True or false?

Lots of people with diabetes get along fine. It's no big deal.
False. Diabetes is a leading cause of devastating kidney failure, heart attack, stroke, blindness, and early death.

If you have a family history of diabetes, you're going to get it, no matter what.
False. You have the power to influence how your genes express themselves. Frequent exercise and good nutrition, along with dietary supplements, can go a long way toward maintaining healthy blood sugar levels for life.

Insulin is the only medical treatment for diabetes.
False. There are a number of pharmaceutical options for treating type 2 diabetes. Furthermore, an exciting new generation of drugs is available to help improve beta-cell function and increase sensitivity to the insulin produced by the body—the two functions that are critical to preventing and treating type 2 diabetes.

Once you develop diabetes, you are doomed to suffer from heart disease, kidney disease, and blindness.
False. In many cases it is possible to dramatically slow down the progression of diabetes or to potentially reverse the course of this disease. You can use an integrative, evidence-based approach that combines innovative new tactics proven effective in five crucial areas—diet, supplements, exercise, lifestyle, and pharmaceuticals.

LEARN HOW TO FIGHT THIS BEATABLE DISEASE WITH . . .
WHAT YOUR DOCTOR MAY NOT *TELL YOU
ABOUT*™ *DIABETES*

"Great guidelines . . . leading-edge information . . . one of the best and most in-depth useful books for people with diabetes . . . This is the right book at the right time to help turn the tide against the growing diabetes epidemic."
—Douglas Kalman, Ph.D., R.D., F.A.C.N., director, Nutrition & Applied Clinical Research, Miami Research Associates

"An entirely innovative guide that offers specific, practical, and attainable measures . . . I recommend it highly to patients and physicians alike."
—Edward P. Hayes, M.D., The Marshfield Clinic, Eau Claire, WI

"An education for the educated patient . . . This book gives solid medical information on diabetes, based on medical studies and solid clinical advice. *I learned a lot from it!*"
—Christopher Cannon, M.D., TIMI Study Group, Boston, MA

"Diabetes is destined to be the scourge of the twenty-first century. As Dr. Joyal states and I concur: 'Diabetes is a disease of accelerated aging.' The link between the two is a destructive biological process known as glycation, which is also a major contributor to cancer, heart disease, Alzheimer's—and even wrinkled, sagging skin. This outstanding book delivers solid science in an exciting and informative format, and provides an excellent program to prevent elevated levels of blood sugar and insulin, thereby enabling us to stop glycation before it starts. Learn how to also help reverse its damaging effects through delicious foods, efficacious nutritional supplements, stress relief, and much more. Highly recommended."
—Nicholas Perricone, *New York Times* bestselling author of *The Wrinkle Cure* and *The Perricone Promise*

"A thoughtful and fresh approach to an old disease of epidemic proportions . . . Dr. Joyal offers new insights and the tools to either avoid or slow down the progression of some of the most basic and aggressive causes of diabetes. An integrated approach to the subject and one you will want to read—now."
—Philip Lee Miller, M.D., author of *The Life Extension Revolution*, and founder, Los Gatos Longevity Institute

WHAT YOUR DOCTOR MAY *NOT* TELL YOU ABOUT®

DIABETES

An Innovative Program to Prevent, Treat, and
Beat This Controllable Disease

STEVEN V. JOYAL, M.D.
with DEBORAH MITCHELL

A Lynn Sonberg Book

GRAND CENTRAL
Life&Style
NEW YORK · BOSTON

PUBLISHER'S NOTE: The information herein is not intended to replace the services of trained health professionals or be a substitute for medical advice. You are advised to consult with your health care professional with regard to matters relating to your health, and in particular regarding matters that may require diagnosis or medical attention.

Copyright © 2008 by Steven V. Joyal, M.D., and Lynn Sonberg
All rights reserved. Except as permitted under the U.S. Copyright Act of 1976, no part of this publication may be reproduced, distributed, or transmitted in any form or by any means, or stored in a database or retrieval system, without the prior written permission of the publisher.

The title of the series What Your Doctor May *Not* Tell You About . . . and the related trade dress are trademarks owned by Grand Central Publishing and may not be used without permission.

Grand Central Life & Style
Hachette Book Group
237 Park Avenue
New York, NY 10017

www.HachetteBookGroup.com

Grand Central Life & Style is an imprint of Grand Central Publishing.
The Grand Central Life & Style name and logo are trademarks of Hachette Book Group, Inc.

The publisher is not responsible for websites (or their content) that are not owned by the publisher.

Printed in the United States of America

First Edition: February 2008
10 9 8 7 6 5 4 3 2

Library of Congress Cataloging-in-Publication Data
Joyal, Steven V.
    What your doctor may not tell you about diabetes : an innovative program to prevent, treat, and beat this controllable disease / Steven V. Joyal with Deborah Mitchell.—1st ed.
      p. cm.
    Includes index.
    ISBN: 978-0-446-69774-3
    1. Diabetes—Popular works. I. Mitchell, Deborah R. II. Title.
    RC660.4.J72 2008
    616.4'62—dc22
                                                                              2007032140

Contents

∞

Introduction

First, the good news: This book presents new, exciting, and most important, safe and effective ways to prevent, reverse, and optimally manage diabetes. We introduce several novel, innovative approaches that, although they are supported by and based on solid scientific research, have been regrettably underutilized, neglected, and ignored for many years.

We say regrettably because—and here's where the bad news comes in—a new study dated June 23, 2007, from the Centers for Disease Control and Prevention (CDC) states that the prevalence of diabetes has been rising 5 percent *per year* since 1990. Millions of people, including an increasing number of young people, are falling victim to this largely preventable metabolic disease every year. As if these statistics were not bad enough, the chief of diabetes surveillance for the Diabetes Program at the CDC, Linda S. Geiss, M.A., recently stated that "this acceleration remains unabated," and that if we want to stop this growing epidemic, "we must improve our prevention efforts."

My experiences in medicine, including my formative years at Dartmouth and Brown medical schools, clinical practice in treating and managing aging patients with type 2 diabetes, years of global responsibility in evaluating pharmaceuticals aimed at treating the root causes of metabolic disease, and invigorating work with leading scientists, has culminated in what I believe to be an optimal strategy for preventing and treating type 2 diabetes. Since 1980, the Life Extension Foundation, where I serve as vice president of scientific affairs, has worked with leading scientists, medical researchers, and nutrition experts to develop innovative, evidence-based disease prevention and treatment approaches and introduce these programs to health-conscious people around the world. In this tradition, _What Your Doctor May_ Not _Tell You About Diabetes_ presents a totally integrated, scientifically based plan to dramatically reduce the risks of metabolic disease and diabetes, from prevention to treatment. This book is a major advance in the prevention, treatment, and risk reduction effort. Here's why.

"Everyone" knows that high blood sugar is the prime killer in diabetes and that it is responsible for blindness (retinopathy), kidney failure (nephropathy), and heart disease. But "everyone" is aware of only half the story. The other half of the story is that a major problem in diabetes is glycation, a nonenzymatic (no enzymes are involved; we will explain this later) process in which sugar molecules attach themselves to protein and lipid (fats) molecules in the body and damage them. Glycation not only devastates vital structures and processes in the body, it is also a key factor in deadly diabetes-related complications, including blindness, nerve damage, and kidney failure, not to mention heart attack and stroke. Glycation also accelerates the aging process.

Of course, controlling blood glucose levels is very important when it comes to controlling the amount of glycation that occurs in the body. However, cutting-edge scientific discoveries reveal that dangerous molecules in our food called glycotoxins (you'll be reading a lot about these damaging substances throughout this book) are also important drivers of lethal glycation reactions. If we want to impact the rising tide of diabetes, prevent new cases from developing, and reduce diabetic complications, then we must be willing to think small—really small. We need to focus on the microscopic yet critical factors that are responsible for the root causes of metabolic dysfunction and diabetes: your molecular makeup and gene expression—that is, how your genes express themselves.

Most often, doctors and patients alike focus on blood sugar alone, without emphasizing that it is the combined problem of insulin resistance and beta-cell dysfunction that is at the root of type 2 diabetes mellitus. Yes, you *can* have a positive impact on the expression of your genes and molecular makeup. Until and unless we address the problems that cause diabetes and metabolic dysfunction in the first place, we will not win our battle.

If it sounds complicated, don't worry. In this book, we tell you exactly what you can do, step-by-step and day by day, to reengineer your body to significantly reduce the risk of diabetes-induced complications (if you already have diabetes) or to prevent diabetes and metabolic dysfunction altogether. We do this by providing proven methods and strategies—no unsafe, pseudoscientific practices or silly (and potentially dangerous) fad diets here.

Mention diabetes, and what are the first things that come to mind? Sugar levels, glucose monitoring, and insulin? If you ask people with diabetes how they manage their disease, they often say, "I watch my sugar" or "I count carbs" or "I take antidiabetes drugs," but I bet you've never heard one of them say, "I'm improving my beta-cell function" or "I'm enhancing my insulin sensitivity." But this is what they *should* be saying and doing if they—and you—want to successfully prevent and treat diabetes. We decided it was time to get the message out, and so we wrote this book to show you how you can use an accessible, integrative, evidence-based method that involves innovative new tactics in five critical areas that are proven to work—diet, supplements, exercise, lifestyle, and pharmaceuticals (if needed)—with details on blood sugar monitoring to reengineer the expression of your body's molecular makeup with the goal of preventing, reversing, and treating diabetes.

This is the first book to bring these five essential elements together in a scientifically based program designed to prevent or treat diabetes. Notice we don't say "steps" because these five areas are *not* steps: you don't do one, then another, and so on. This is an *integrative approach; these elements complement each other.*

The book's format is easy to follow. In part I, we introduce the new concepts mentioned earlier and how they relate to the overall picture of diabetes and more important, how understanding them will help you achieve your goals. Included in this discussion is a detailed look at diabetic complications and how knowledge of these new concepts will help you avoid or alleviate these problems.

In part II, we look at the five essential elements of our diabetes program, dedicating a chapter to each element, with two chapters for the critically important nutritional component. We begin, however, with a detailed look at how we screen for and diagnose diabetes—how mainstream medicine has largely been underutilizing several effective tools and how our approach works best to identify prediabetes and diabetes and thus better identify risk early on, when our evidence-based approach can have the greatest impact. We conclude part II with stories from real diabetes patients and a wealth of resource information that you can start to use today to live a healthier, happier, longer life.

The road to prevention and effective treatment begins here. Don't walk—get ready to run with us!

PART I

The Real Story of Diabetes

Chapter 1

It's in Your Genes

glycation - the bonding of a sugar molecule to a protein or lipid molecule without enzymatic regulation.

Diabetes is a serious disease and an ever-growing epidemic that can be reversed and prevented if you think really small. We're talking about the realm of genes and molecules, where mainstream medicine is just beginning to put to good use the hard-earned knowledge gained from other scientific disciplines like molecular biology and nutritional science. We know that if you think about and act on the small stuff, you can get huge results: the vast majority of cases of type 2 diabetes can be prevented altogether or treated much more effectively if you use all the tools at your disposal.

Our approach is to target the three features of the disease (we call these the "Big Three" of diabetes) that many people have heard little or nothing about: beta-cell function and insulin resistance (also known as impaired insulin sensitivity, a hallmark of not only type 2 diabetes but also metabolic syndrome), and a biological process called glycation, which we will explain

3

in greater detail shortly. We believe it is critical not only that you understand these three concepts but that you—indeed, everyone who is touched by diabetes or is at risk of metabolic disease—adopt the strategies we know will positively impact the Big Three. Our goal is to prevent diabetes or, if you already have the disease, greatly enhance your quality of life and alleviate the impact of potentially deadly diabetic complications.

How can you achieve these goals? The journey begins with your molecular makeup. Despite what you may believe, it is not inevitable that you will develop diabetes, be obese, have high blood pressure, or have a heart attack (or a second heart attack) just because you have a family history and it's "in your genes." You have the power to influence how your genes express themselves—that is, how they contribute to various biochemical reactions that occur in your body. In fact, everyday activities and situations can dramatically influence your gene expression—exercise, weight loss, the types of foods you eat, the use of dietary supplements and/or pharmaceuticals, stress—all of these factors influence how your genes express themselves.

We'll begin in this chapter with a basic introduction to diabetes, where we explain what's happening at the cellular level—specifically beta-cell function and insulin resistance (an inability of the body's cells and tissues to increase their intake of glucose [blood sugar] in response to the insulin that is circulating in the bloodstream), which are critical factors in the prevention and better management of diabetes.

Wait, you may be thinking, isn't control of blood glucose levels the key to diabetes management?

In fact, elevated blood glucose levels are a *sign* of an underlying problem, not the *key* to the problem. The combination of beta-cell failure and insulin resistance is responsible for type 2 diabetes. If you focus on enhancing beta-cell function, increasing insulin sensitivity, and controlling glycation, you can dramatically change the course of type 2 diabetes or even prevent it altogether.

DIABETES: THE BASICS

Diabetes is, unfortunately, a relatively common disease, and many people either know someone who has the condition or have it themselves. Therefore, it's easy to fall into the trap of thinking diabetes "isn't a big deal." I actually overheard someone express that very sentiment during a recent scientific conference. Such thoughts stem from the fact that most people know very little about the disease or its devastating impact on the body, and even many doctors don't fully understand the core causes of the disease.

In this chapter, we will provide you with a clear understanding of the basic causes of diabetes, including an eye-opening look at the link between premature aging and diabetes. First, however, we will begin with a brief introduction to what precedes the diagnosis of diabetes—prediabetes (technically referred to as *impaired fasting glucose* [IFG] or *impaired glucose tolerance* [IGT], but for simplicity's sake, we will refer to these interrelated conditions as prediabetes). Although we discuss prediabetes in greater detail in the next chapter, it is important to have a general idea of what this condition is before we dive into our discussion of diabetes.

Prediabetes is a condition in which a person's blood sugar levels are above normal but below the level required for him or her to be (technically) diagnosed with frank (or full-blown) diabetes. This condition affects approximately 16 percent of Americans and in many people develops into full-blown type 2 diabetes over the course of ten years—therefore the term "prediabetes." The two most important messages we need to emphasize at this point regarding prediabetes are (1) prediabetes is preventable and much easier to reverse than frank diabetes (and please know that type 2 diabetes is not an inevitable result of prediabetes), and (2) prediabetes is often accompanied by other symptoms, such as obesity and high blood pressure, that significantly and independently increase your risk of developing other serious medical conditions, including heart attack and stroke.

With that brief introduction out of the way, let's turn to you. The vast majority of people fall into one of four categories when the topic of diabetes arises, and chances are you do, too:

- You want to prevent diabetes. You don't have signs or symptoms of the disease, but you recognize how serious the disease is and you want to help ensure you never get it. Congratulations for being proactive and forward thinking!
- You have prediabetes. This is the best time in the course of metabolic disease to reverse its direction and restore your metabolic health. Remember, if you take action now, you can prevent type 2 diabetes quite easily.
- You have diabetes. Just because you have diabetes doesn't mean you can't significantly improve your health and adopt habits that can dramatically reduce your risk of developing complications. Furthermore (and this is most exciting), we have had great success with many people in this category who have completely weaned themselves (with their doctors' guidance) from antidiabetes drugs by following the program described in this book.
- You have a family member or friend who has the disease and want to find ways to help that person better manage and control the metabolic complications. We can help.

DIABETES IS A FORM OF ACCELERATED AGING

Why do we begin a discussion of diabetes with this statement? Because we want to get your attention; because it's true; because very few people realize or know about the interesting connection between accelerated aging and metabolic disease (including diabetes); and because we want to motivate you to take action *today* to prevent or reverse prediabetes or to better manage diabetes and prevent diabetic complications. No one wants to age any faster than he or she has to, and the information we share with you in this book has the added potential benefit of helping to slow down the aging process.

The link between diabetes and accelerated aging is a process called *glycation,* a common chemical reaction in which a sugar molecule is bonded to a protein or fat molecule inside the body (endogenous glycation) or outside the body (exogenous glycation). Limiting glycation is critical when it comes to preventing, reversing, or treating diabetic complications. The process of glycation and the resulting production of cell-damaging substances called advanced glycation end products (AGEs) and advanced lipoxidation end products (ALEs), both of which are known collectively as *glycotoxins,* are a major focus of this book, and they are terms that will soon become very familiar to you. What is disturbing is that despite the very strong scientific evidence that glycation is a crucial factor in diabetes-related complications and premature aging, there is virtually no discussion of these factors in most publications on diabetes.

UNDERSTANDING METABOLISM: BLOOD SUGAR AND INSULIN

Diabetes is a disease that is characterized by abnormal metabolism, so our discussion begins with a look at how metabolism works in healthy individuals. "Metabolism" refers to the processes by which the body breaks down and builds up substances for use by the cells, although it is the breakdown of food, and its transformation into energy, that is most often associated with the word. Of the three types of nutrients (proteins, carbohydrates, fats) metabolized by the body for energy and growth, carbohydrates and fats are the primary sources of energy.

Carbohydrates (sugars and starches) are broken down into smaller sugar molecules (glucose) in the intestinal tract and then enter the bloodstream, where they circulate and wait to be transported into cells so they can be used to provide energy. But these sugars can use some help to enter cells, and that assistance comes in the form of a hormone known as *insulin*. Insulin is produced in the pancreas by specialized cells called *beta cells*. The most important function of insulin is to facilitate the passage of glucose into cells, which means it also helps regulate blood glucose levels. Insulin also plays a major role in how the body uses amino acids to build proteins, and it helps stimulate growth and tissue development by preventing the abnormal breakdown of proteins, fats, and the storage form of glucose, called glycogen.

Beta cells can sense the amount of glucose in the blood. When they sense that blood glucose levels are rising, which occurs after eating, they secrete more insulin into the bloodstream so it can signal, for example, muscle cells to "take up" glucose (allow glucose to enter the cell through the cell membrane). Insulin's signal to cells to take up glucose from the bloodstream causes blood sugar levels to fall. As blood sugar levels fall, beta cells reduce their production of insulin. This is how the process works in healthy people.

But for millions of Americans—approximately 54 million, according to the latest data from the National Institute of Diabetes and Digestive and Kidney Diseases (NIDDK)—abnormalities in their metabolism herald diabetes. Let's take a brief look at this most common of all metabolic diseases.

TYPES OF DIABETES

Approximately 21 million Americans have diabetes, according to the Centers for Disease Control and Prevention (CDC), and more than twice that number have prediabetes and are at risk for the disease. The somber statistics from the American Diabetes Association show that the majority of people with prediabetes will develop type 2 diabetes within ten years if they do not take steps to include dietary and exercise changes to prevent it. Given that more than 60 percent of Americans are overweight (body mass index [BMI] of 25 or greater) and nearly one third of them are obese (BMI of 30 or greater), and that a growing percentage of young people are overweight as well, it is projected that there will be a 165 percent increase in the number of people with diabetes by 2050. It is also projected that without preventive efforts, one third of the children born in the year 2000 will develop diabetes in their lifetime.

There are two major types of diabetes—type 1 (formerly called juvenile-onset diabetes or insulin-dependent diabetes) and type 2 (formerly called adult-onset diabetes or non-insulin-dependent diabetes). (See "Signs and Symptoms of Diabetes," page 10.) Both are the result of a dysfunction in metabolism that causes abnormally high levels of glucose to accumulate in the bloodstream. In type 1 diabetes, which usually develops during childhood or early adolescence, the pancreas does not produce insulin. Therefore, those with the disease must take insulin every day for the rest of their lives. This form of diabetes affects about 5 percent of those who have the disease and is currently believed to be autoimmune in nature, which means the body produces antibodies that destroy its own cells; in this case, the beta cells. The exact cause is unknown, although genetic factors, environmental influences, diet, and viruses are all being closely explored as contributing factors.

SIGNS AND SYMPTOMS OF DIABETES

Signs and symptoms can include the following:

- frequent urination
- excessive thirst
- increased fatigue
- unusual/unexplained weight loss
- irritability
- blurry vision
- frequent infections of the skin, urinary tract, or vagina
- poor wound healing
- tingling in the hands or feet

Note: In some cases, people with prediabetes have some of these signs and symptoms. If dangerously high blood sugar levels develop suddenly, additional symptoms may include acetone-scented breath or body odor; abdominal pain; nausea; vomiting; low blood pressure; slow, deep breathing pattern; and a reduced level of consciousness.

In type 2 diabetes, which affects around 90 percent of people who have diabetes, the body still produces insulin, but the process is dysfunctional: the beta cells of the pancreas cannot produce and secrete the amount of insulin required by the body (decreased beta-cell function results in decreased insulin secretion), and the body becomes less sensitive (more resistant) to the effects of insulin. Indeed, insulin resistance is a key underlying factor in type 2 diabetes and a topic we will discuss in depth.

Since type 2 diabetes is by far the most common form of diabetes and is the type that commonly arises after the warning signal of prediabetes, we will focus on this disease. You can also prevent, and in many cases reverse, type 2 diabetes because the disease is largely influenced by the collective impact of diet, exercise, and other lifestyle practices on gene expression of metabolism. One of the advantages of type 2 diabetes is that it develops gradually over time, and the body typically offers some clues and indications that the disease is in your future *if* you don't take measures to prevent it.

Both type 1 and type 2 diabetes share the unfortunate ability to cause devastating long-term complications that can affect nearly every organ system in the body, including the eyes, kidneys, heart, and nerves, and can ultimately result in kidney failure, blindness, amputations, heart disease, and stroke. This is a critical point to understand, as many people have the misconception that only people who have type 1 diabetes are at risk for these complications as they grow older. Nothing could be further from the truth. *Everyone* who has diabetes, whether type 1 or type 2, is at risk. In fact, even people who have prediabetes are at risk for heart attack and stroke, so it is never too early to take aggressive preventive measures.

Type 2 Diabetes in Children and Adolescents

The label "adult-onset" once used to describe type 2 diabetes no longer applies, as more and more young people develop this form of the disease. The statistics are grim. In 1992, the presence of type 2 diabetes among children was uncommon, but by 1994, up to 16 percent of new cases were being diagnosed in urban pediatric centers. By 1999, that percentage had grown to between

WHO HAS DIABETES?

Prevalence Among U.S. Population 20 Years and Older (adjusted for population age differences)

- Men: 10.5%
- Women: 8.8%
- People 60 years or older: 20.9%
- American Indians/Alaskan Natives: 19%
- Non-Hispanic blacks: 15.7%
- Hispanics/Latinos: 14.8%
- Non-Hispanic whites: 8.7%

SOURCE: CDC National Diabetes Fact Sheet: www.cdc.gov/diabetes/pubs/pdf/ndfs_2005.pdf; 2005 estimates are taken from 1999–2002 NHANES estimates of total prevalence projected to 2005, also on the CDC Web site.

8 and 45 percent, depending on the area of the country surveyed. Most of the newly diagnosed cases of type 2 diabetes among young people in the United States are among African American, Mexican American, and Native American children. Along with ethnicity, the primary risk factor is obesity, accompanied by a lack of physical activity. Other risk factors for childhood development of type 2 diabetes include a family history of the disease, puberty, female gender, and being born to a mother who had diabetes. It is *especially critical* that we reverse the progression of the disease in children and adolescents, because the presence of the disease exposes them to additional decades of damage from elevated blood glucose levels and glycation.

Preventing, Reversing, and Treating Diabetes

One of the problems with how type 2 diabetes is addressed and treated today is that few people—including physicians—take into consideration the differences between early and advanced stages of the disease. During the early stages, people typically have hyperglycemia (high blood sugar levels) and hyperinsulinemia (high blood insulin levels), and the logical therapeutic approach is to increase insulin sensitivity and improve beta-cell function. Yet too often physicians prescribe oral antidiabetes drugs made with "old" technology, which raise insulin levels in the blood regardless of blood sugar levels. The use of drugs that indiscriminately raise insulin levels is not ideal. These old-technology drugs are called sulfonylureas, and we discuss them in more depth in chapter 10.

Our approach to the treatment of prediabetes and early-stage type 2 diabetes is to improve insulin resistance and beta-cell function through an integrated, scientifically sound program that includes the following:

- a power-packed yet short-duration exercise program (How does a whopping twelve minutes every other day sound to you?)
- a unique yet incredibly simple nutrition plan that does not involve deprivation or fad dieting
- a nutraceutical supplement plan based on published scientific studies that naturally supports healthy blood sugar levels
- cutting-edge pharmaceuticals (if needed) to restore damaged insulin-producing beta cells and improve insulin sensitivity

NEW WAYS TO LOOK AT DIABETES

We want you to get used to several new ways of looking at diabetes, ways that we are almost certain you have not heard discussed but that are fundamental to understanding, preventing, and managing the disease, as well as enhancing quality of life and longevity in people with type 2 diabetes.

Tame Your Gene Expression

Foremost is an idea we mentioned previously: that you can dramatically influence how the genes involved in glucose metabolism are expressed. Although you can't change your genes, you can change the degree of expression of your genes. This means that you can impact to what degree certain genes involved in blood sugar metabolism are turned on or off. In fact, you can easily and conveniently modify the expression of your genetic code through lifestyle modifications, including food choices, exercise, stress management, and the use of botanicals, nutraceuticals, and medications (if needed). All of these choices are explained in part II of this book.

Getting At the Core Issues

We also want you to understand that the key to preventing and managing the core causes of type 2 diabetes is improving beta-cell function and addressing insulin resistance. The high blood sugar that is found in type 2 diabetes is a *sign* of the actual causes of the disease. Although it is true that it is important to carefully track and monitor blood glucose levels, a better way to think about type 2 diabetes is to focus on modifying the core causes of the disease—namely, beta-cell dysfunction and insulin resistance. A clear understanding of these two features of diabetes and how to manage them effectively are especially crucial when we look at the big picture of diabetes, prediabetes, and metabolic syndrome.

(In the interest of clarity, we would like to note that prediabetes and metabolic syndrome are often thought to be the same thing, but they are not. While the main diagnostic criterion for prediabetes is a fasting blood sugar level between 100 and 126 mg/dL or a two-hour postprandial [after eating] blood sugar level of 140 to 199 mg/dL as of this writing, metabolic syndrome uses a similar defining blood sugar level as well as several other defining factors, including blood pressure, lipid/cholesterol levels, and waist circumference. However, both prediabetes and metabolic syndrome share a common factor—insulin resistance.)

Three Components of an Optimal Prevention and Management Plan

Prediabetes is at epidemic levels: according to the latest information from the NIDDK, approximately 54 million Americans have prediabetes, and the majority of these people will develop diabetes eventually unless they make lifestyle changes.

We believe that there are three key components of an optimal plan to prevent and manage diabetes. These components are interrelated, and are therefore prime examples both of the complexity of diabetes and of the amazing way various body systems work together. They are:

- insulin resistance and beta-cell dysfunction and how they relate to diabetes. A core understanding of this relationship is often lacking in people who have diabetes and it is often not explained by physicians to their patients.
- oxidative stress, which has a devastating impact on both metabolic and cardiovascular function in people who have prediabetes or diabetes.
- glycation, AGEs (advanced glycation end products), and ALEs (advanced lipoxidation end products), known collectively as glycotoxins, which can cause irreversible damage in people with diabetes. Glycation is a core factor in diabetic complications.

Diabetes Is a Form of Accelerated Aging

The fact that diabetes is a form of accelerated aging is a surprise to most people. Yet over decades of research, scientists have been uncovering the root causes of premature aging. We know that in both aging and diabetes, two important biological processes occur that result in damage to the body: *glycation,* which results in damage to protein and lipid molecules, and *oxidative stress,* characterized by increased free-radical activity and damage to tissues by molecules like reactive sugar aldehydes.

Research shows that life expectancy for people with diabetes is four to eight years less than for people without diabetes. Diabetes and aging share many signs and symptoms in common, too, including:

- skin conditions, such as infections, thin skin, rashes, and discoloration
- loss of elasticity and flexibility of skin and other tissues
- cardiovascular ailments, including heart attack, poor circulation in the legs, atherosclerosis (a general term for several diseases characterized by thickening and hardening of the arteries), and stroke
- increased prevalence of certain types of cancer (pancreas, colon, liver)
- vision problems, including cataracts, glaucoma, and retinal degeneration
- hearing loss
- impotence
- memory loss or other cognitive impairment

Given that diabetes and aging share so many characteristics, it's not surprising that they also respond to many of the same interventions, as we discuss in chapter 8.

INSULIN RESISTANCE

The term "insulin resistance" is not usually mentioned when doctors speak to their patients about optimal diabetes management. Because the term often confuses patients (and physicians, too, on occasion), we will take time to explain exactly what it means.

Insulin resistance is an impairment of the body's ability—specifically the liver, fat, and muscle cells—to use insulin to process glucose (sugar). As a result, glucose isn't handled properly by the body, and blood sugar levels rise. In the early stages of insulin resistance, the body recognizes that blood sugar levels are elevated, so the beta cells try to step up the secretion of insulin to overcome this cellular resistance. This places stress on the pancreas until, over time, the pancreas becomes dysfunctional and unable to produce enough insulin to help control blood sugar levels. The vast majority of individuals with type 2 diabetes are also insulin resistant, as are many people who have high blood pressure and/or cardiovascular disease, and who are overweight or obese.

All people with metabolic syndrome have insulin resistance—in fact, insulin resistance is likely the key cause of the constellation of findings observed with metabolic syndrome. More than twenty years ago, Gerald Reaven, M.D., of Stanford first coined the term "Syndrome X" to describe the constellation of signs and symptoms caused in certain patients by insulin resistance, including high blood sugar levels, high blood pressure, cholesterol and lipid abnormalities, and an increase in waist circumference. He continues to research this condition to this very day.

Not everyone who is insulin resistant goes on to develop diabetes. In fact, if you discover you are insulin resistant, you can take steps to help reverse the condition. In the recent past, you would have needed to undergo complicated, expensive, and time-consuming tests at academic medical centers to identify whether you were insulin resistant. Today, however, commonly available blood tests allow us to identify those who have or who are at high risk for insulin resistance, as we discuss in chapter 4 in detail.

Causes of Insulin Resistance

We know that insulin resistance runs in families and certain high-risk ethnic groups (such as Pima Indians); therefore, genes play a role in its development. Being overweight or obese also is a contributing factor, because excess fat impairs insulin sensitivity. Insufficient exercise also reduces the ability of muscles to use insulin. Many people who have insulin resistance and high blood sugar have at least one or more of the following conditions: high triglyceride levels (a type of fat in the blood), high blood pressure, low high-density lipoprotein (HDL) blood levels (the "good" cholesterol), and/or excess abdominal girth (a "beer belly"). This combination of conditions is known collectively as metabolic syndrome or insulin resistance syndrome. We'll talk much more about insulin resistance and its interrelationship with prediabetes and diabetes in chapter 2.

Lighten up and chill out! Research has shown that insulin resistance is associated with stress, hostility, and high cynicism. A 2006 study published in *Psychosomatic Medicine* reports that people with high levels of hostility typically have worse insulin resistance when they are experiencing stress, especially high levels of chronic stress. It is possible that stress-reduction methods may help in this context (see chapter 9).

How to Prevent or Reverse Insulin Resistance

The good news is that there are effective, easy-to-adopt ways to change the course of insulin resistance at the cellular level. These include lifestyle modifications, such as making optimal nutritional choices that will ultimately change gene expression involved in glucose metabolism, learning new ways to prepare foods, learning the optimal way to exercise, using natural supplements and, if needed, using pharmaceuticals. All of these options are discussed in depth in part II of this book.

OXIDATIVE STRESS

Oxidative stress is a condition in which the body is subjected to an excessive number of highly reactive molecules known as *free radicals*. Recall from high school chemistry that molecules are composed of atoms, which in turn each consist of a nucleus, protons, neutrons, and electrons. The atoms of a molecule are held together by chemical bonds, which are controlled by the electrons. When these bonds are broken—which occurs naturally as part of metabolism, for example—free radicals are produced. The body can often ward off the damage these free radicals may cause by sending in *antioxidants,* substances that prevent the *oxidative* damage free radicals can inflict on the body's tissues. (We discuss antioxidants and their value in diabetes prevention in chapter 8.)

If, however, the body is under stress, which can be caused by a failure to follow a diet that contains sufficient amounts of antioxidants (in other words, lots of fresh fruits and vegetables), the body may not be capable of neutralizing these damaging molecules. Exposure to environmental toxins (pollution, food additives, radiation, pesticides, and cigarette smoke, for example) stimulates the production of free radicals. If the body is unable to neutralize free radicals, the end result may be damage to the body's cells, tissues, and organs. This damage has been associated with several complications of diabetes, including injury to the heart and blood vessels. In addition, free-radical damage is a well-known cause of the accelerated aging of tissues in the body.

Oxidative Stress and Diabetes

Although there are many different types of free radicals, the ones that play an especially critical role in causing cardiovascular problems in people with diabetes include the superoxide radical and peroxynitrite. Research has shown that hyperglycemia (high levels of glucose in the blood) promotes the formation of free radicals, and therefore oxidative stress as well. In particular, hyperglycemia can cause excess production of superoxide. Oxidative stress, in turn, stimulates the development and progression of diabetes and the complications associated with it. Other situations that promote oxidative stress in prediabetes and diabetes include:

- hyperinsulinemia (elevated insulin levels)
- elevated fasting and postmeal (postprandial) levels of triglycerides and cholesterol stress
- elevated levels of superoxide, which in turn generate highly reactive peroxynitrite and can trigger many damaging events in the body, including heart, kidney, blood vessel, and eye problems
- repetitive episodes of ischemia (lack of blood flow and oxygen to tissue), which occurs in diabetes patients who have coronary artery disease (CAD) and peripheral vascular disease

Oxidative stress can impair insulin activity in several possible ways. Some research even suggests that oxidative stress can serve as a key initiating trigger for diabetes. Sophisticated experiments on insulin resistance show that repeated exposure of insulin-resistant tissue to oxidative stress can result in hyperglycemia.

How to Reduce Oxidative Stress in Diabetes

Currently, studies are investigating the use of antioxidants to stave off the development or continuance of oxidative stress in people with diabetes. In chapter 8, we will explore that research and discuss which antioxidants may be most effective for you. Other studies may also prove helpful. Researchers in Japan, for example, found that patients with type 2 diabetes and disease of the teeth and gums (known as periodontal disease, which is very common in people with diabetes) who underwent periodontal therapy experienced a reduction in oxidative stress. These and other methods to reduce oxidative stress are covered in part II of this book.

GLYCATION AND GLYCOTOXINS AGE YOU FASTER

When we tell patients that glycation is one of the major consequences of diabetes and a contributing factor in diabetes complications, the typical response is, "I've never heard of it. Is it something new?" When we tell them that scientists have known about glycation since at least 1912 and of its major impact on diabetes and diabetic complications since the 1980s, the typical response is, "Why haven't I heard about it? Why isn't my doctor talking about it?"

Glycation is a biochemical process that involves a series of nonenzymatic reactions (those that don't require enzymes to make them happen) between proteins and/or certain lipids (fats) and glucose that result in the development of the toxic substances we mentioned earlier, AGEs—advanced glycation end products—and ALEs—advanced lipoxidation end products. If you've ever made toast, then you've experienced glycation firsthand. Toasting bread involves the Maillard reaction, named after the French chemist who investigated this chemical reaction in the early years of the last century. The Maillard reaction is the browning reaction that occurs when food is heated and cooked at high temperatures. This reaction is also commonly observed when we grill lamb chops, make French fries, and broil salmon steaks.

Levels of AGEs and ALEs increase as people grow older, and those levels are fueled by the foods they eat. In the past, scientists were not fully aware of the impact of food-derived glycotoxins on human cells, organs, and tissues. However, recent groundbreaking research has uncovered startling evidence of the very important role that food-derived glycotoxins play in contributing to glycation in the body. Furthermore, AGEs play a major role in the aging process as well as in diseases such as diabetes, heart disease, kidney disease, cancer, Alzheimer's disease, and certain types of neuropathy. Our primary focus is on the relationship of AGEs and ALEs to diabetes and complications of the disease. For the sake of simplicity, we will refer to AGEs and ALEs collectively as glycotoxins throughout the book.

Glycotoxins and Diabetes

The role of glycotoxins in diabetes is especially significant. Because they are a key factor in complications associated with diabetes, it has become increasingly clear that we need to understand how glycotoxins are formed, how to prevent their formation, and how to reduce their negative impact on health.

Glycotoxin levels increase dramatically in people who have elevated blood glucose levels, because these substances thrive in high-glucose environments. Thus, glycotoxins are especially prevalent in individuals who have prediabetes or diabetes. Sites in the body especially susceptible to the accumulation of glycotoxins include the renal glomerulus (in the kidney), the retina (the membrane at the back of the eye that helps you see), and important blood vessels like the coronary arteries (the arteries that supply blood to the heart). We also know that glycotoxins play a significant role in causing chronic diseases that are associated with underlying inflammation, such as heart disease and neuropathy.

How Glycotoxins Are Formed in Food

Food-derived glycotoxins are formed during a series of chemical reactions that take place between glucose and the proteins, lipids, and nucleic acids derived from the food you eat. These reactions ultimately damage tissues in the body, as glycotoxins prompt cells to send messages that lead to the production of inflammatory substances called cytokines. Experimental studies show that this is exactly what happens in glycotoxin-caused vascular (blood vessel) damage often seen in diabetes.

Hemoglobin A_{1c} (Hb A_{1c}) is an advanced glycation end product (AGE) that is created when glucose molecules bind to hemoglobin, a protein in blood. Measurement of this factor in the blood is very helpful in monitoring the level of glycation damage in prediabetes and diabetes. We discuss several surprising facts about Hb A_{1c} in chapter 4.

An important strategy to reduce the level of glycation damage to your tissues is to keep your blood glucose levels within a healthy range (below 100 mg/dL premeal or after a fast, although we know from our extensive research in this area that fasting blood sugar readings in the 70 to 85 mg/dL range appear optimal). We talk about how you can achieve this goal throughout part II of this book.

Glycotoxins are also formed during food production and preparation. Food manufacturers use various heating processes to enhance flavor, color, and texture; to improve food safety (sterilization and pasteurization); and to extend shelf life. A by-product of these processes, unfortunately, is often glycotoxins. Foods as varied as cola drinks, infant formulas, baked goods, caramel, and brewed products contain glycotoxins. Foods high in fat and protein (such as meat and poultry) typically have the highest glycotoxin levels. How you prepare your food (or have it prepared for you if you eat out) can also have a signifi-cant impact on the formation of glycotoxins. We discuss the amount of glycotoxins in various foods in detail in chapter 5, on nutrition.

If blood glucose levels remain high and/or your diet contains high amounts of glycotoxins, your tissues will become inflamed. Glycotoxins are especially harmful to people with diabetes, as these toxic molecules are associated with retinopathy (glycotox-ins accumulate in the retinal blood vessels), neuropathy (they accumulate in peripheral nerves, resulting in nerve damage), kidney failure (they are found in kidney tissue), heart disease, and blood vessel disease. The use of antiglycotoxin agents or in-hibitors, such as aminoguanidine, has been studied in the hope of preventing or reversing diabetic complications triggered by high levels of glycation/glycotoxins. We discuss these and other measures in chapter 8.

How to Avoid Glycotoxins in Your Diet

Research strongly indicates that cooking foods rich in protein, fat, and fructose (a common sugar found in many foods, both naturally and/or as an additive) at high temperatures greatly increases the formation of glycotoxins, while cooking foods with liquid, such as steaming, poaching, braising, and stewing, at temperatures less than 250°F reduces glycotoxin formation. A great many foods contain glycotoxins; in fact, food manufacturers have been adding glycotoxins to their products for many years as a cheap way to enhance flavor and appearance. The dramatic increase in processed foods in recent years and the fact that fast food has become a staple of the American diet mean that most people are consuming unprecedented amounts of food-derived glycotoxins. A high-fat diet clearly enhances glycation.

Cutting-edge research shows that restricting dietary glycotoxins in people with diabetes results in a significant reduction in substances that indicate inflammation; namely, C-reactive protein (CRP) and peripheral mononuclear cells, and tumor necrosis factor alpha (TNF-alpha). Excess inflammation in the body is a serious health risk that demands immediate attention. Therefore, in our detailed discussion of food and diabetes in chapters 5 and 6, you will learn how to avoid dietary glycotoxins and the best ways to prepare foods to prevent their formation.

Yet another way to deal with glycotoxins is through the use of pharmaceuticals. Research suggests that at least two types of drug classes currently available, angiotensin II receptor blockers (ARBs) and angiotensin-converting enzyme inhibitors (ACE inhibitors), which are commonly prescribed to people who have diabetes and/or hypertension, help protect against glycotoxin-induced kidney damage. You can read more about this topic in chapter 10, on the use of pharmaceuticals in diabetes.

INFLUENCING GENE EXPRESSION

You inherited your genes (a set of coded information in the form of DNA) from your parents. Although your genes were set at birth and don't change during the course of your lifetime, what many people don't realize is that literally everything you do as well as everything you are exposed to in your environment influence the *expression* of your genes. That means your genes are expressed—literally turned on and turned off—by what you eat and how much, your level of physical activity, your use of nutraceuticals and/or pharmaceuticals, and the level of stress you encounter every day and how you cope with it. You have control over all of these factors, which means you can make changes in your lifestyle that can impact your genes in a meaningful way that will enhance your health.

Have you ever heard the expression "You are what you eat"? Well, there's a great deal of truth to this statement. For example, omega-3 fatty acids have a favorable impact on the genes involved in metabolism. These essential fats, found in fish oil, flaxseed, and walnuts, positively affect genes that code for proteins critical to cholesterol metabolism and body weight regulation.

The Influence of Nutrition on Gene Expression in Metabolism

We know that what you eat influences the expression of genes involved in glucose metabolism. For example, research shows that eating a diet including a moderate amount of carbohydrates rich in soluble fiber and adequate amounts of "good fats"—monounsaturated fats and essential fatty acids—is a good nutritional strategy for helping to positively influence the expression of several genes contributing to insulin resistance and systemic inflammation.

You can also target specific genes, gene factors, and biochemical functions in your battle against elevated glucose levels and metabolic dysfunction. We know, for example, that a genetic factor called carbohydrate-responsive element binding protein (ChREBP) regulates glucose metabolism in the liver. Two nutrients known to directly influence this genetic factor are docosahexaenoic acid (DHA) and eicosapentaenoic acid (EPA), essential fatty acids that are found in relatively high concentrations in fish like salmon, mackerel, sardines, and tuna. (These nutrients are also available as dietary supplements, which may be preferable because of the contaminants—mercury, cadmium, polychlorinated biphenyls [PCBs], dioxins, and others—that pollute much of the world's seafood supply. High-quality supplements can be purchased that have had these toxins removed.) Technically speaking, DHA and EPA down regulate the gene expression of ChREBP, which results in better glucose control.

Nutraceuticals also can influence gene expression. Cinnamon extracts, for example, can be helpful in controlling glucose levels, as can barley extracts, which appear to work similarly to the antidiabetes drug metformin. These and many more examples of nutraceuticals that can help you influence the expression of your genes are discussed in chapter 8.

THE BOTTOM LINE

We introduced a lot of information in this chapter, but the take-home message is this: If you want to prevent, reverse, or better manage diabetes and its complications, you need to focus on and better understand the core causes of the disease itself and the cause of diabetes-induced damage—beta-cell dysfunction, insulin resistance, and glycation/glycotoxins. You need to address the first two factors to help you correct the underlying cause of type 2 diabetes, and you need to learn how to minimize the impact of the third factor to reduce the risk of developing complications from diabetes. We'll begin by looking at two conditions that precede and/or coexist with diabetes: prediabetes and metabolic syndrome.

Chapter 2

Prediabetes and Metabolic Syndrome

In 2002, at least 54 million Americans—52 million adults and 2 million adolescents—had prediabetes—a condition that puts them on the fast track for developing type 2 diabetes and all of the serious lifestyle and medical complications associated with the disease. Unfortunately, not only does the number of people with prediabetes continue to rise, but the problem is now becoming common among young people, corresponding with the rising number of overweight and obese children and adolescents.

Piggybacking on the epidemic of prediabetes is a closely associated condition—metabolic syndrome. As we mentioned in chapter 1, it is possible to have prediabetes and not have metabolic syndrome, but the truth is that most people who have prediabetes or diabetes have characteristics that are consistent with metabolic syndrome as well.

A cluster of conditions that increase the risk of heart disease, stroke or diabetes

29

THE METABOLIC SYNDROME CONTROVERSY

Some experts have argued that the diagnosis of metabolic syndrome is artificial, because the core defect of metabolic syndrome is also shared with type 2 diabetes and prediabetes—insulin resistance. In fact, Gerald Reaven, M.D., who coined the term "Syndrome X" to describe the constellation of findings seen in insulin-resistant patients, recently argued this point. Reaven stated in the June 2006 edition of the *American Journal of Clinical Nutrition* that the World Health Organization, the Adult Treatment Panel III, and the International Diabetes Federation have all created diagnostic criteria for metabolic syndrome, but that diagnosing the syndrome in a person isn't nearly as important as targeting the core underlying problem—insulin resistance—and aggressively taking steps to reduce the risk of heart disease and stroke in these people. We agree.

The methods outlined in this book can help you reverse, prevent, or more effectively treat insulin resistance, a core defect of metabolic syndrome as well as prediabetes and diabetes. In this chapter, we'll begin by giving you a clearer understanding of how insulin resistance operates in the body, which will, in turn, give you a better idea of how to make the best use of the intervention strategies discussed in part II of this book.

PREDIABETES

Charlene is a forty-year-old marketing executive living in Manhattan who had grown to hate her job and wanted to make a career move. The stress of looking for a job while trying to maintain her hectic work schedule was wearing her down and causing her to experience heart palpitations, so she made an appointment to see her doctor. Although she said she knew she could "stand to lose more than a few pounds," she was somewhat surprised when her doctor told her she had high blood pressure and that her fasting blood glucose level was "in the high prediabetes range." He urged her to lose weight and recommended she talk with a diabetes educator. Knowing she had a history of heart disease and diabetes in her family, Charlene took the news from her doctor as a wake-up call.

"I didn't really think hard about it until the next day," says Charlene. "But the day after my doctor told me about my high blood pressure and prediabetes, I was sitting in the office of a huge marketing company, and the interviewer asked me where I saw myself in ten years. Suddenly I realized that unless I made some lifestyle changes, I would probably have diabetes and heart disease within ten years. Both my parents are overweight, and both have diabetes. My older brother has heart disease. I couldn't even think about the job right then; all I could do was think that I might not have a future—not with that company, or with my kids or my family."

Studies suggest that most people who have prediabetes develop type 2 diabetes within ten years unless they lose 5 to 7 percent of their body weight (that's 10 to 15 pounds if you weigh 200 pounds). Because the vast majority of people with prediabetes are overweight or obese, the recommendation we make that they introduce modest changes in their diet and amount of physical activity can help them achieve their weight loss goals as well.

How Prediabetes Is Diagnosed

Prediabetes is a condition in which either a person's fasting blood glucose level or two-hour postprandial (after eating) blood sugar level is higher than normal but lower than the threshold for a diagnosis of diabetes. Most doctors today use one of two tests to detect prediabetes: the fasting plasma glucose test (FPG) or the oral glucose tolerance test (OGTT). The FPG measures glucose in blood that is drawn after a ten- to twelve-hour overnight fast; the OGTT measures glucose after a similar fast and then again two hours after drinking a glucose drink.

In addition to these two tests, there are two other equally easy-to-administer tests that check for the level of glycation that is occurring in the body and identify those individuals at high risk for the damaging consequences of excess glycation. We discuss these often-overlooked tests in depth in chapter 4.

Prediabetes is diagnosed if the fasting blood glucose level is from 100 to less than 126 mg/dL (below 100 mg/dL is considered to be normal). A reading greater than or equal to 126 mg/dL is defined as diabetes. For the OGTT results, a reading of 140 to 199 mg/dL two hours after drinking the glucose drink indicates prediabetes (a reading less than 140 mg/dL is considered to be normal).

I am among a group of health-care professionals who believe that an ideal fasting plasma glucose reading is between 70 and 85 mg/dL. In 1999, research showed that fasting blood sugar levels in excess of 85 mg/dL were associated with an increased risk of heart disease.

Charlene was offered the job at the management consulting firm, and one of the perks of the job was membership at a health club.

We don't know whether Charlene has followed through on the advice of her doctor and is regularly using the health club, but she would certainly be wise to do so. Studies show that people with prediabetes can prevent or delay the development of type 2 diabetes by up to 58 percent if they make modest changes to their lifestyle—basically diet and exercise modifications—that result in a weight loss of 5 to 7 percent. The dietary and exercise recommendations we explain in this book, consistent with the latest innovations in evidence-based medical science, can significantly improve that percentage and put you back on the road to health.

A diagnosis of type 2 diabetes has the potential to gravely and adversely impact the life of anyone who receives it, especially since few people think ahead or realize they are in danger because usually, like Charlene, they have no symptoms. This is one of the major problems with prediabetes: it is essentially a silent condition. The defining characteristic of prediabetes is an elevated blood glucose level, and that can be identified only through a blood test (see chapter 4). Because prediabetes is an insidious condition that progresses slowly over years, many people are surprised when, after getting a fasting blood glucose test, their doctors tell them they have type 2 diabetes. "How did that happen?" they often ask. The usual way—slowly and progressively over time. Identifying prediabetes allows people an opportunity to take steps to significantly reduce the risk of developing type 2 diabetes.

Risk Factors, Signs, and Symptoms: Prediabetes

Like most people who have prediabetes, Charlene is overweight. And although people with prediabetes typically don't experience strong symptoms, at least during the early years of progression—when interventions can have the most powerful impact on reversing the course of the disease—there are risk factors you should consider. They include the following:

- being overweight or obese
- having a sedentary lifestyle (little or no regular exercise)
- having a family history of diabetes, especially parents and/ or siblings
- having given birth to a baby who weighed more than 9 pounds

Prediabetes in Young People

Because more and more young people are being diagnosed with type 2 diabetes, we believe it is *critical* that we recognize and address the problem of prediabetes (as well as insulin resistance) among children and adolescents. Similar to adults, we can reverse the trend toward type 2 diabetes in young people if we identify those at greatest risk and act early. If your child has any one of the first three risk factors listed above, especially if he or she is overweight or obese, it is important that he or she be screened for elevated blood sugar levels (see chapter 4 for detailed testing information).

METABOLIC SYNDROME

As mentioned in chapter 1, metabolic syndrome is a constellation of risk factors for cardiovascular disease caused by insulin resistance. Experts estimate that about 25 percent of Americans have signs and symptoms characteristic of metabolic syndrome.

The exact criteria required for a diagnosis of metabolic syndrome differ somewhat among about a half dozen organizations, including the World Health Organization; the American Heart Association; and the National Heart, Lung, and Blood

Institute. For discussion purposes, we will use the definition put forth by the Third I   ort of the National Cholesterol Education Program Expert Panel on Detection, Evaluation and Treatment of High Blood Cholesterol in Adults. This definition states that a diagnosis of metabolic syndrome should be given when someone has three or more of the five characteristics named below. Having just one of the characteristics increases your risk of heart disease, and having at least three of them increases your risk even more. The five characteristics are:

- excess body fat around the waist: for men, 40 inches or greater; for women, 35 inches or greater
- elevated triglyceride levels: equal to or greater than 150 mg/dL
- reduced good cholesterol (high-density lipoprotein [HDL]) levels: less than 40 mg/dL for men; less than 50 mg/dL for women
- elevated blood pressure: equal to or greater than 130/85 mm Hg without antihypertensive medication
- elevated fasting glucose levels: equal to or greater than 100 mg/dL

Two other risk factors that we feel are important to mention but are not commonly included are (1) the presence of a high level of fibrinogen and/or plasminogen activator inhibitor-1 in the blood (two blood clotting factors associated with an increased risk of coronary heart disease) and (2) an elevated level of C-reactive protein in the blood, which is an indication of inflammation and one of the elements for which we strongly recommend testing (see chapter 4). In 2001, for example, there were several studies indicating that high levels of fibrinogen are also a significant risk factor for stroke.

Excess Abdominal Body Fat

Research shows that having fat around the abdomen (often referred to as an "apple shape" or a "beer belly"), and not just total body fat, is associated with insulin resistance and an increased risk for heart disease. The risks associated with the accumulation of excess fat around the abdomen have been known for some time. In 2005, researchers published the results of a study that followed 27,270 men for thirteen years. During that time, 884 men developed type 2 diabetes. Compared to men with the smallest waists (29–34 inches), men with larger waists were at least twice as likely to develop diabetes, and those with the largest waists (40 inches or greater) were up to twelve times more likely to develop diabetes.

Triglycerides

Triglycerides are a type of fat that is stored primarily in fat tissue and, to a lesser degree, circulates in the bloodstream. High levels (greater than 200 mg/dL) of triglycerides in the blood are often associated with diabetes and an increased risk of heart attack. (See chapter 4 for information on triglyceride testing under "Lipid Test.")

Although triglycerides are fats, an important dietary factor that influences their level in the bloodstream is carbohydrate. A diet that contains a high level of certain carbohydrates, especially simple sugars like fructose, causes triglyceride levels to rise, while a more moderate intake of carbohydrates (see chapters 5 and 6), along with exercise and the use of supplements as needed, can help optimize triglyceride levels and increase beneficial HDL in the blood.

High-Density Lipoprotein Cholesterol

High-density lipoprotein (HDL) is the "helpful" (think "H" = "high" = "helpful") lipid-protein compound because it aids in eliminating excess cholesterol from the vascular system and reduces the risk of heart and blood vessel diseases. As with triglycerides, you can improve your HDL levels by making modifications to your diet, especially by including healthy fats (such as monounsaturated fats and omega-3 fatty acids), avoiding trans fats (discussed in chapters 5 and 6), exercising, drinking only moderate amounts of alcohol (one to two glasses of red wine daily is acceptable), maintaining a healthy weight, and not smoking. You may be surprised, for example, that something as simple as adding walnuts to your diet each day can improve your HDL levels. Indeed, walnuts are just one of the foods that favorably modify gene expression.

Blood Pressure

"If I hadn't gone to that health fair with my neighbor, I probably still would not know that I have high blood pressure," says Ellie, a forty-eight-year-old nursery school teacher. "I hadn't been to see my doctor in several years because I didn't have a reason to go, so I didn't think anything was wrong." But the 165/95 mm Hg reading Ellie got at the health fair came as an unwelcome and unexpected surprise and was incentive enough for her to heed the advice of the nurse who took her pressure to make an appointment with a doctor.

An estimated one-quarter of American adults have high blood pressure (hypertension), which is defined as 140/90 mm Hg or higher in nondiabetics. Blood pressure that remains between 120–139/80–89 mm Hg is considered to put people at risk for hypertension, although these defined values are changing as more evidence accumulates about the very real dangers of even relatively small increases in blood pressure. Recall that a blood pressure of 130/85 mm Hg or greater is one of the parameters for metabolic syndrome.

For people with diabetes, most medical societies recommend that patients try to reach a target blood pressure of less than 130/80 mm Hg, which reflects the increased risk of heart disease in diabetes patients. We recommend that blood pressure be (ideally) less than 120/80 mm Hg.

Ellie's situation is not unusual; because hypertension is a silent disease—meaning it typically has no symptoms—it often goes unnoticed. The danger of undetected high blood pressure is that it makes the heart work too hard and in turn increases the risk of many serious and life-threatening conditions, including stroke, atherosclerosis, congestive heart failure, kidney disease, heart disease, and blindness. According to the National Heart, Lung, and Blood Institute, about two-thirds of people older than sixty-five have high blood pressure. The time to take steps to avoid or reverse high blood pressure is now. The steps outlined in part II of this book tell you how.

RISKS ASSOCIATED WITH INSULIN RESISTANCE

The risks associated with insulin resistance are considerable and include diabetes, heart disease, stroke, polycystic ovary syndrome, fatty liver disease, nonalcoholic steatohepatosis (fatty inflammation of the liver), and sleep apnea. The risk of developing these conditions can be significantly reduced if you take the steps outlined in part II of this book. Compared with people who do not have insulin resistance, people with this problem are exposed to increased cardiovascular risk.

In a study of men without cardiovascular disease, those who had three or more features of insulin resistance (metabolic syn-

BLOOD PRESSURE IN A NUTSHELL

- The first number is the systolic pressure, which is the force of blood in your arteries as your heart beats. For people who are fifty years or older, the systolic number gives the most accurate diagnosis of hypertension.
- The second number is the diastolic pressure, which is the force of the blood in the arteries as the heart relaxes between beats.
- You do not need to have an abnormally high diastolic pressure in order to have high blood pressure—a high systolic reading is enough to warrant a diagnosis of hypertension. This condition is called isolated systolic hypertension, which is a common form of hypertension among aging Americans.
- Generally, systolic blood pressure increases with age.
- Optimal blood pressure can often be achieved successfully without the use of medication by following the guidelines offered in part II of this book. When necessary, medications can be added to your other treatment strategies.

drome) at the beginning of the investigation had more than twelve times the risk of developing cardiovascular disease and more than six times the risk of developing type 2 diabetes by the end of the study, seven years later. Other studies show that death from cardiovascular disease increased by 60 to 280 percent, and death from coronary heart disease increased by 70 to 330 percent in people who have insulin resistance/metabolic syndrome.

HOW TO AVOID OR TREAT INSULIN RESISTANCE/ METABOLIC SYNDROME

The strategy to reduce the risks associated with insulin resistance and metabolic syndrome includes many of the same strategies you should take to avoid diabetes:

- Know your body composition—measure your waist (greater than 40 inches for men and greater than 35 inches for women means increased risk) and work toward or maintain a healthy body weight.
- Incorporate regular exercise into your life to help reduce body fat and the associated increased risk of heart disease and other complications from being overweight.
- Take the steps necessary to correct high blood pressure, low HDL levels, and high triglyceride levels.

In the second part of this book, we provide you with innovative, easy-to-follow nutritional information and recipes, exercise guidelines, and the latest information on how to incorporate nutritional supplements into your prevention or treatment program to optimize your metabolic health.

METABOLIC SYNDROME/INSULIN RESISTANCE: RISING RISK IN CHILDREN AND ADOLESCENTS

Although the conditions that characterize metabolic syndrome/ insulin resistance traditionally have been seen in aging adults, more and more often they are appearing in young people. This is a highly disturbing trend, as these life-threatening health problems have the potential to carry over into adulthood and cause significant risks throughout life unless they are reversed and managed early.

Thirteen-year-old Madison "has always been a big girl," says her mother, Tracy. "She was nearly ten pounds when she was born, and since my husband Rich and I are not thin, we just accepted the fact that she was going to be big." When it was time for Madison to attend summer camp, however, a required medical examination revealed that she had high blood pressure and high cholesterol. Tracy was shocked.

"I always thought high blood pressure and high cholesterol only affected older people," she said. "Suddenly the doctor is telling us that our daughter could develop heart disease. Heart disease! I decided then and there that we had to do something about this, and that it was going to have to be a family effort."

Madison is fortunate that her parents decided to take action, which in their case included a total makeover of their diet and planned regular exercise. Their daughter's condition also prompted Tracy and Rich to have their own health evaluated, and they found that they, too, had high blood pressure, high cholesterol, and prediabetes. Despite some reluctance on Madison's part, Tracy and Rich were able to help their daughter, and themselves, lose weight and bring down their blood pressure and cholesterol levels over a period of eight months.

"We're still not at our goal weight," said Tracy, "but Madison is actually doing better than we are. We're helping each other."

In a study published in 2004 in the *New England Journal of Medicine,* researchers studied 470 obese and overweight children and adolescents of various ethnicities and compared them with their non-obese peers. As the level of obesity increased, so did the prevalence of metabolic syndrome, which reached 50 percent among the most severely obese youngsters. Levels of C-reactive protein also were high in the youngsters, and all of the overweight and obese children already had signs of cardiovascular disease.

These findings are not unique, and in fact many subsequent studies have reported similar shocking results and disturbing statistics. A 2006 study from Children's Hospital in Boston compared the prevalence of metabolic syndrome in twelve- to nineteen-year-olds in the National Health and Nutritional Examination Survey (NHANES) from two time periods: 1988–1994 and 1999–2000. The researchers found that metabolic syndrome affected 9.2 percent of young people in the earlier survey and 12.7 percent in the later one, and that the increase was due mainly to an increase in body weight. Overall, 38.6 percent of overweight or obese youngsters had metabolic syndrome, compared with 1.4 percent of normal-weight young people. Along with the conditions associated with metabolic syndrome, these youngsters also had higher C-reactive protein levels, which are an additional risk for cardiovascular problems.

Besides being overweight or obese, several other risk factors are associated with metabolic syndrome among young people. If, for example, you are a woman who has diabetes and you have a child who weighed more than 9 pounds at birth, your child is at significant risk of developing metabolic syndrome in childhood and diabetes later in life. Research also shows that infants with lower birth weights whose mothers were obese but not diabetic at the time they gave birth are also at increased risk of developing metabolic syndrome. Given that more and more children and adolescents are overweight and obese, these findings are a warning that the combination of obesity and metabolic syndrome will continue to be a serious problem unless we take action. As a mother, father, or other individual who is responsible for a child's health and welfare, you need to help protect and preserve the future health of your child.

THE BOTTOM LINE

An understanding of insulin resistance is important if you are to successfully prevent, reverse, or treat the conditions it causes. In this chapter we impressed upon you the interrelationship between insulin resistance, prediabetes, and metabolic syndrome and the value of blood testing for early diagnosis. We also want to stress the value of blood tests to assess the level of glycation occurring in your body. You will learn much more about these tests and the impact of glycation on premature aging and diabetic complications in future chapters.

Next, we'll turn our attention to a topic that is on the mind of everyone who has or who is at risk for diabetes: complications. Although having diabetes changes your life, it is the development of complications from diabetes that can cause truly devastating, life-altering events.

Chapter 3

Complications of Diabetes

The complications of long-term elevated blood sugar levels and runaway glycation wreak havoc with the human body. In diabetes, complications include blindness; loss of toes, feet, or legs; kidney failure; as well as a much greater risk of certain cancers, heart attack, and stroke. In fact, for those patients with diabetes who do little or nothing to reduce the risk of these complications, diabetes-related problems are a near certainty, not a theoretical possibility. The good news is that you can take steps *today* to ensure a future without diabetic complications or one in which the risk of developing the devastating complications of diabetes is greatly minimized.

When discussing the complications associated with diabetes, two major hurdles come to mind, both of which we explore in this chapter. One is that there is little emphasis placed on the driving factors behind the damage caused by diabetes, including glycation and the work of free radicals and oxidative stress, which we touched on in chapter 1. We know that both of these factors have a major role in the deadly complications associated with diabetes. That's why we cannot emphasize strongly enough that if we do not aggressively target interventions aimed at reducing these destructive processes, your ability to win the battle against diabetes complications will be compromised.

The other major hurdle is that although diabetes patients fear complications, too many hold on to the idea that the problems will happen to other people, not to them. Whenever my colleagues and I discuss the grave importance of aggressively treating the disease with diabetes patients or with the general public, the attitude that "well, this will happen to someone else, not me" is all too common. The stark truth, however, is that diabetes is a relentlessly progressive disease, and given enough time, complications are a virtual certainty among patients with poorly controlled diabetes *unless* aggressive steps are taken to reduce the risk.

In this chapter, we briefly explore the seriousness of diabetic complications and explain how glycation, oxidative stress, and other factors are responsible for their development. We also share with you how an integrated, evidence-based approach that combines an antiglycation diet, exercise, natural supplementation, lifestyle modifications, and pharmaceuticals (when indicated), along with appropriate blood glucose testing and monitoring, allows you to dramatically reduce many risk factors that lead to complications from diabetes. We also refer you to appropriate chapters in the second part of the book where you can get the practical, step-by-step guidelines you need to fight and win the battle against diabetic complications.

THE CHALLENGE OF COMPLICATIONS

Diabetic complications can affect many parts of the body and cause a variety of symptoms, yet one characteristic they share is that they develop over time. Complications from diabetes seed, take root, and develop over ten, fifteen, twenty years or longer, depending on many factors, such as the severity of the elevated blood glucose, the person's age, the degree of damage caused by glycotoxins, the level of oxidative damage, the presence of other health problems, and what steps, if any, have been taken to alleviate or treat these issues.

Damage to your eyes, nerves, kidneys, and blood vessels due to diabetes begins to develop very early in the course of the disease and is accelerated if you do not take aggressive steps to control your blood glucose levels, oxidative damage, and the level of glycation occurring in your body. Even if you have diabetes complications right now, you can still do many things to dramatically minimize or halt further damage.

The results of two landmark studies provide strong evidence that this is true. The Diabetes Control and Complications Trial (DCCT) showed that people with type 1 diabetes can reduce their risk of developing diabetic complications by 50 percent or more if they take aggressive measures to control their disease, while the United Kingdom Prospective Diabetes Study (UKPDS) revealed that people with type 2 diabetes can also enjoy significant reductions in the risk of complications if they are diligent about making changes in their treatment as the disease progresses. Although the results of the UKPDS point to the importance of controlling blood sugar to reduce complications from the disease, the program in this book provides a far greater, more multifaceted strategy proven to work by targeting other key factors (such as oxidative stress and glycation) to achieve significant risk reduction.

Diabetes complications fall into two main categories: macrovascular and microvascular. Macrovascular complications involve the heart and major blood vessels and can lead to heart attack and stroke. Microvascular complications involve small blood vessels and damage the eyes, kidneys, skin, and nerves throughout the body, resulting in neuropathy, vision problems, infections, and kidney disease. Let's take a look at some of the sobering statistics.

Microvascular Complications

- Diabetes is the leading cause of kidney failure, representing 44 percent of all new cases in 2002.
- About one-third of diabetes patients have severe periodontal disease, resulting in damage to the teeth and gums.
- Sixty to 70 percent of people with diabetes have nervous system damage, which can have wide-ranging effects throughout the body.
- Diabetes causes 12,000 to 24,000 new cases of diabetic retinopathy (damage to the delicate light-sensing membrane, the retina, of the eye) each year.
- Male diabetics are twice as likely to have sexual dysfunction as males who don't have diabetes.
- Diabetes is the leading cause of new cases of blindness among adults aged twenty to seventy-four.
- People with diabetes are nearly twice as likely to get glaucoma as other adults.
- Diabetes patients are twice as likely to get cataracts as people without diabetes. Cataracts also develop at an earlier age among people who have diabetes.
- Skin and urinary tract infections are more common among men and women who have diabetes.
- More than 60 percent of nontraumatic amputations of

the lower limbs are performed on people who have diabetes. In 2002, for example, about 82,000 such amputations were required for people with diabetes.

Macrovascular Complications

- Adults with diabetes have heart disease death rates that are two to four times greater than adults who don't have diabetes.
- The risk for stroke is two- to fourfold higher among people with diabetes.
- Among newly diagnosed type 2 diabetics, the risk of stroke within five years of diagnosis is 100 percent greater than that of the general population, according to a study published in *Stroke* in 2007.
- Studies suggest that more than 70 percent of people with diabetes have blood pressure that is greater than or equal to 130/80 mm Hg or are taking antihypertensive medication.

The critical take-home message is not only that these complications are a significant concern if you have diabetes, but also that the seeds of these problems are planted very early in the disease process. Indeed, in many cases, the complications associated with diabetes, such as damage to the blood vessels, nerves, kidneys, and skin, begin to occur before the disease is officially diagnosed, which again highlights the need for early diagnosis and aggressive treatment.

CARDIOVASCULAR DISEASE: ENDOTHELIAL DAMAGE

The link between diabetes and cardiovascular disease (conditions that affect the heart and/or large blood vessels: heart disease, peripheral vascular disease, and stroke) is well established and hard to ignore: nearly 80 percent of people who have diabetes die from heart and/or blood vessel diseases. The risk of developing cardiovascular problems usually begins many years before diabetes is diagnosed; that is, when prediabetes and/or metabolic syndrome are present.

A key factor in the increased risk of cardiovascular disease seen in patients with long-term, poorly controlled diabetes is endothelial dysfunction. The endothelium consists of a delicate layer of cells that line the blood vessels. Damage to endothelial cells is a key initiating event in atherosclerosis. (As mentioned earlier, atherosclerosis is the most common type of arteriosclerosis, a general term for several diseases characterized by thickening and hardening of the arteries.) Some of the dysfunction is related to aging; with the passing years, the endothelial cells are less able to renew themselves, and the barrier layer weakens. In addition, the scientific literature reveals that atherosclerosis is associated with insulin resistance/high levels of blood sugar and insulin; elevated levels of C-reactive protein, low-density lipoprotein (LDL), and triglycerides; as well as low levels of high-density lipoprotein (HDL) and testosterone.

For example, a recent clinical study in patients with type 2 diabetes showed the dramatic negative impact of a meal rich in glycotoxins on endothelial function and oxidative stress. After ingesting a meal high in dietary glycotoxins, the patients experienced severe impairment of both macrovascular and microvascular function. They also showed increased indications of endothelial dysfunction and oxidative stress.

A major study highlights the increased risk of cardiovascular disease in type 2 diabetes. In the Nurses' Health Study, in which investigators observed the incidence of heart disease, stroke, and type 2 diabetes among 117,629 female nurses over a twenty-year period, the study researchers found that women who eventually developed type 2 diabetes had a fourfold greater risk of having a heart attack and a twofold greater risk of stroke than women who did not develop diabetes. As you now know, the culprit behind these complications is insulin resistance fueled by glycation/dietary glycotoxins, and oxidative stress. Not surprisingly, the study's investigators also found that increased weight gain was significantly associated with a greater risk of cardiovascular disease among women with diabetes.

INFLAMMATION, GLYCOTOXINS, CARDIOVASCULAR DISEASE, AND DIABETES

Glycotoxins interact with advanced glycation end product–(AGE–) binding receptors, a process that leads to a major feature of cardiovascular disease and diabetes—vascular inflammation, or inflammation of the blood vessels. Vascular inflammation begins very early in people who have insulin resistance. Glycotoxins accumulate in the vascular tissues, especially in the tissues of people who have high blood glucose levels, and play a key role in the formation and growth of atherosclerotic lesions by causing damage to the vascular endothelium. In atherosclerosis, damage to the endothelium triggers a cascade of inflammation resulting in an accumulation of plaque (fats, cholesterol, and other substances) in the arteries that supply the heart (which leads to coronary artery disease), the brain (responsible for stroke), or the legs (responsible for the poor circulation that can lead to diabetic foot infections and, ultimately, amputations of the lower extremities). Atherosclerosis can also affect the arteries that supply the kidneys.

Although atherosclerosis can affect people who don't have diabetes, we know the disease progression is greatly accelerated in people who have diabetes and is two to six times more likely to develop in diabetes patients than in those without the disease. Glycotoxins also can alter low-density lipoprotein (LDL) cholesterol and cause it to stick to blood vessel walls, causing a buildup of plaque and "hardening of the arteries."

More Cardiovascular Complications

Although high blood glucose is a major player in heart and blood vessel diseases, the interaction of glucose with other risk factors also significantly increases the risk of potentially fatal cardiovascular disease. Let's take a brief look at each of these factors.

- **Hypertension.** According to one study, 71 percent of patients with diabetes have high blood pressure, 29 percent of diabetics do not know they have hypertension, and 43 percent of diabetics who have hypertension are not being treated for it. Separately, diabetes and high blood pressure are risks for the development of atherosclerosis. When they occur together, the risk of heart attack, stroke, and kidney disease increases dramatically.

- **Low HDL.** Levels of HDL lower than 40 mg/dL if you are male or lower than 50 mg/dL if you are female are associated with an increased risk of cardiovascular disease. HDL transports cholesterol away from the arteries and back to the liver so it can be eliminated from the body and helps remove cholesterol from plaque in the blood vessels.

- **High triglycerides.** Elevated levels of this form of fat typically are seen along with low HDL cholesterol. This combination of abnormal lipid levels is very common in people who have diabetes and who are obese or physically inactive. High triglyceride and low HDL levels are important risk factors for ischemic stroke (stroke that occurs due to a blockage of blood flow to the brain) among people who have heart disease. Many people are not aware that elevated triglyceride levels alone increase your risk of heart attack nearly threefold.

- **Obesity.** Obesity increases the risk of cardiovascular disease and premature death. It is also a proinflammatory condition, which means that excess adipose (fat) tissue releases substances such as inflammatory cytokines and other factors that are associated with insulin resistance, elevated blood pressure, and oxidized cholesterol (which promotes the formation of plaque), all of which are implicated in heart disease and stroke.

A recent study that looked at more than 172,000 individuals found that the risk of heart attack or death was 78 percent higher among people who had metabolic syndrome than among those who did not. The study's main author and colleagues emphasized that the increased risk ranged from 50 to 200 percent, with greater risk among women.

How to Reduce the Risk of Cardiovascular Complications

To prevent, reduce, or minimize the risk of cardiovascular complications, consider the following strategies, all of which are discussed in detail in the second part of this book:

- Incorporate a regular exercise program into your lifestyle. We make specific, time-sensitive recommendations in chapter 7. How does twelve minutes a day sound to you?
- If you are overweight, lose weight. (There are no silly and unscientific fad diets in our program, just an innovative, easy-to-follow nutrition plan that minimizes food-derived

glycotoxins without causing feelings of deprivation and an exercise program that is unbelievably brief. This special approach is described in chapters 5, 6, and 7 to help you with this important goal.)

- Incorporate nutritional supplements scientifically shown to help optimize cardiovascular health (see chapter 8).
- If you smoke, quit. (Don't despair—it takes, on average, at least seven tries to eventually stop smoking! Keep at it—hypnosis, support groups, acupuncture, and recently approved medications can help you quit the habit. You'll get there!)

KIDNEY DISEASE

An important, often overlooked factor in the development of diabetic kidney disease is the damage caused by glycation (damage arising from both high blood sugar levels and dietary glycotoxins). In fact, glycotoxins from the diet play a major role in glycation-induced damage in kidney failure, according to important research. The study shows that restricting the amount of glycotoxins in the diet leads to reduced levels of these damaging substances in the bloodstream, which in turn reduces glycation-induced damage in the kidneys.

How Kidney Damage Occurs

When kidneys function normally, they filter toxins from the blood and maintain a healthy balance between water and salts in the body. Your kidneys also help regulate red blood cell levels and manufacture hormones that help regulate your blood pressure. When blood glucose, glycotoxins, and oxidative stress are elevated, kidney function begins to deteriorate. Once diabetes-induced kidney damage begins, you need to aggressively reduce the rate of damage in order to prevent the development of end-stage kidney disease in diabetes. End-stage disease occurs when the kidneys operate at 10 percent or less of their capacity. Those with this complication need dialysis or a kidney transplant in order to survive.

One of the first signs of kidney damage is the presence in the urine of a protein called albumin, which can be detected through an analysis of a urine sample (a urinalysis). If this early stage of kidney damage (called microalbuminuria, the presence of small amounts of albumin in the urine) is not detected or treated, the kidneys will increasingly lose their ability to function, and levels of a substance called creatinine will increase in the blood. Creatinine is an indicator of the kidneys' filtering ability. A creatinine level greater than 1.5 mg/dL is considered abnormal, but if blood pressure and blood glucose levels are controlled with diet, exercise, supplements, and medications—including angiotensin II receptor blockers (ARBs) and angiotensin-converting enzyme inhibitors (ACE inhibitors) (discussed in chapters 5 through 10), it is possible to halt further damage and/or dramatically reduce the progression of the disease.

Kidney failure is characterized by an abnormally low glomerular filtration rate. The glomeruli are sieve-like structures in the kidney that process blood and filter out waste products, fluid, and various other substances. When glycotoxins damage kidney cells, the glomeruli lose their ability to filter the blood properly, allowing toxins, excess fluid, and other products to build up in the body. A glomerular filtration rate greater than 90 milliliters per minute indicates normal function; 60 to 90 indicates a mild decrease in function; 30 to 59, moderate; 15 to 29, severe. Less than 15 is a diagnosis of kidney failure. Because chronic kidney disease typically develops over many months or years, it is important to regularly check your kidney function, especially if you have diabetes.

A study (*Journal of the American Society of Nephrology,* January 2007) showed that diabetes patients who are obese (especially those with excess fat around the abdomen) are at increased risk of developing kidney disease. The patients were part of the landmark Diabetes Control and Complications Trial (DCCT), which showed that intensive control of diabetes significantly reduces the risk of kidney disease and other diabetic complications. In this analysis, the risk of kidney disease was 65 percent less among patients who were on intensive therapy versus those on conventional therapy.

How to Prevent Kidney Damage

Once kidney cells are damaged, they cannot be repaired. But you can prevent further damage and dramatically slow progression of the disease. Here's how.

• Keep glycation and free-radical damage at bay. This means you need control blood sugar levels by following an antiglycation eating program, supplementing with appropriate nutraceuticals, and taking appropriate diabetes medication. (See part II for details on these recommendations.)

• Keep your blood pressure well controlled, preferably around 115/75 mm Hg, and speak with your doctor about possibly taking ACE inhibitors or angiotensin II receptor blocker antihypertensive drugs. These medications can help control blood pressure, reduce microalbuminuria, and reduce glycation.

• Beware of urinary tract infections. These infections are common in people with diabetes and can severely damage the kidneys. Therefore, at the first sign of a urinary tract infection (fever, chills, flank pain, suprapubic pain [pain in the central lower abdomen, above the pelvis], frequent urination, burning when urinating, cloudy or bloody urine, feeling the constant urge to urinate), see your doctor immediately.

• Get your creatinine and albumin levels checked. The presence of microalbuminuria suggests early kidney damage, and an elevated creatinine level can be a sign that your kidneys are beginning to deteriorate. (Please note: an elevated creatinine level can also be seen in dehydration and in people who have high levels of muscle mass, among other situations.)

DIABETIC NEUROPATHY

Diabetic neuropathy is the result of nerve damage caused by chronically elevated blood sugar levels, glycation, and free-radical stress/oxidation. Numbness, pain, and muscle weakness are typical characteristics and usually occur in the lower extremities, but diabetic neuropathy can have devastating effects elsewhere in the body as well.

Diabetic neuropathy is usually divided into four categories—peripheral, autonomic, proximal, and focal. Let's take a brief look at each of them.

Peripheral Neuropathy

The foot is the body part most commonly affected by peripheral diabetic neuropathy. Peripheral neuropathy can also affect the legs, arms, and hands. The nerve damage may first appear as discomfort, tingling, extreme sensitivity to touch, loss of coordination or balance, numbness, or the sensation of getting needle pricks and may graduate to severe pain or cramps followed by the disappearance of the pain and/or numbness. Disappearance of the pain can indicate that the nerve cells have been irreparably destroyed, and in this situation your extremity is insensitive to touch and pain. Although the lack of pain is a relief, it also leaves you with an increased risk of developing potentially deadly complications, including life-threatening infection. This is why people with diabetes must check their feet for scrapes, cuts, swelling, bleeding, and signs of infection every day if they have peripheral neuropathy. I recall a middle-aged patient several years ago who developed a very serious foot infection after she stepped on a nail. She had long-standing diabetic peripheral neuropathy in her feet due to poor blood sugar control and runaway glycation, and she did not feel the nail go into her foot. Poor circulation, which is also common among people with diabetes, increases the risk of developing nonhealing foot ulcers.

Left untreated, an infection can spread to the bone and result in the need for amputation of the affected toes, foot, or lower leg. About half of the more than 82,000 lower limb amputations performed in the United States each year are for people with diabetic neuropathy. The tragedy of amputation can be prevented in many cases if more attention is paid to the first signs of infection in the feet (see "Caring for Your Feet," page 58).

Sensory neuropathy can also result in muscle weakening or wasting (amyotrophy). If the nerve cells responsible for stimulating certain muscles are destroyed, the muscles decrease in strength and size. A condition called foot drop, for example, develops when the nerve cells responsible for stimulating the muscles that raise the foot are destroyed. The result is that your foot slaps the floor every time you take a step. With rehabilitation, this condition can be improved. Femoral neuropathy, which is seen in some people who have type 2 diabetes, begins as pain in the front of the thigh. As the nerve cells are destroyed, muscle weakness and wasting follow, and it can become difficult to lift your leg, climb stairs, or rise from a seated position.

CARING FOR YOUR FEET

- Clean your feet every day using warm (not hot) water and mild soap. Dry your feet, especially between your toes.
- Inspect your feet daily for cuts, blisters, redness, swelling, or other problems. You can use a mirror to see the bottoms of your feet, or ask someone else to check them for you.
- Always protect your feet by wearing shoes or slippers. Wear seamless socks to avoid irritating your feet.
- Keep your toenails short and clean. Nails should be cut to the shape of your toes and filed with an emery board. Be very careful not to cut or damage your skin—infection can result.
- See a podiatrist *very frequently.*
- Do not wear tight or ill-fitting shoes. You should be able to move your toes when standing in your shoes.

Autonomic Neuropathy

Autonomic neuropathy affects the nerves that are associated with the function of various organs and organ systems, including the heart, blood vessels, digestive system, urinary tract, reproductive organs, sweat glands, and eyes. Autonomic neuropathy can cause hypoglycemia unawareness, in which people are unable to sense the warning signs and symptoms of hypoglycemia (low blood sugar). (See chapter 10 for more on hypoglycemia unawareness.) Some of the more common conditions associated with autonomic neuropathy in people with diabetes include the following.

- **Gastroparesis.** The vagus nerve is the main nerve responsible for moving food through the digestive tract. If this nerve is damaged by glycation and free-radical damage/oxidation as well as other elements associated with long-term exposure to glucose, the intestinal and stomach muscles can stop working properly, and food will move much more slowly through the digestive tract. This condition is known as gastroparesis. Because the stomach of someone who has gastroparesis does not empty itself normally, it is more challenging to monitor and control blood glucose levels. Symptoms of gastroparesis include early fullness (feeling full after eating very small amounts of food), nausea, vomiting of undigested food, abdominal bloating, and weight loss.

- **Cardiovascular problems.** Nerve damage to the cardiovascular system affects how the body makes adjustments to blood pressure and heart rate. For example, damage to the nerves that control blood pressure may cause blood pressure to fall rapidly after people stand and can result in fainting (a condition known as orthostatic hypotension).

- **Neurogenic bladder.** When nerve cells in the bladder are damaged, the bladder is often prevented from emptying completely, which allows bacteria to grow in the bladder and kidneys, resulting in urinary tract infections. An inability to recognize when the bladder is full or to control the muscles that release urine are also possible results of nerve damage to the bladder.

- **Reduced sexual response.** Both men and women may experience a reduction in sexual function, although neuropathy does not change sex drive per se. Men most often experience erectile dysfunction, while women may have problems with arousal, orgasm, or lubrication.

• **Vision problems.** Nerve damage to the eyes can make the pupils less responsive to light, which has negative effects on how people see at night or in any dark environment (see "Retinopathy and Other Vision Problems" in this chapter).

Proximal Neuropathy

Proximal (or lumbosacral plexus) neuropathy affects the nerves in the thighs, hips, and buttocks, usually on one side of the body only. The nerve damage causes weakness and pain in the legs that typically worsen as the condition progresses, making it very difficult for people with the neuropathy to rise from a seated position without assistance. Unexplained weight loss is another common characteristic of this neuropathy.

Focal Neuropathy

Focal neuropathy is an often unpredictable and painful condition in which specific nerves, usually in the head, torso, or legs, become painful and/or weak. Symptoms may include paralysis on one side of the face (Bell's palsy), double vision, eye pain, or severe pain in one area, such as the leg, chest, or lower back. This form of neuropathy is not particularly common in diabetic neuropathy, but it can occur.

Prevention and Treatment of Diabetic Neuropathy

There are several important steps you need to take to prevent and treat diabetic neuropathy.

• Limit glycation-induced nerve damage by controlling blood sugar levels.

- Reduce food-derived glycotoxins by adopting an antiglycation eating plan (see chapters 5 and 6).
- Incorporate the use of nutraceuticals and (if necessary) medications to fight glycation and oxidative stress.

We discuss these steps in detail in part II.

RETINOPATHY AND OTHER VISION PROBLEMS

The eyes and the blood vessels that supply them with nutrients and oxygen are among the most sensitive areas of the body, so it's no surprise that elevated blood glucose levels can have a significant impact on eye health. In fact, vision problems, including damage to the retina, glaucoma, and cataracts, are very common among people who have chronically high blood sugar levels and diabetes.

Gregory, a sixty-one-year-old landscape foreman, was diagnosed with type 2 diabetes at age fifty-six. He said he took "reasonably good" care of himself when it came to exercise, but his diet "could stand some improvement." He also admitted that he had not had an eye examination in nearly three years, a situation that changed shortly before his last birthday, when he began to notice blurry vision. Fearing the worst, he made an appointment with his ophthalmologist, who told him that the lenses of both eyes were affected by his elevated blood sugar levels and that improved blood sugar control could remedy the situation. Gregory, although upset about his vision, was pleased that he could take steps to control the situation.

"I'd been lax in controlling my glucose," he says, "and I didn't want to pay for it by losing my sight." Gregory immediately began to watch his diet much more closely and test his blood glucose at least twice a day. By the end of three months, the blurry vision had disappeared, and his glucose levels had improved significantly. Gregory was thrilled.

"It just goes to show you the power of the fork," he says. "I don't want to lose my sight because I refuse to make a few diet changes. It's absolutely not worth it."

Gregory was fortunate, as blurred vision can also be a sign of other, more serious eye problems, such as retinopathy, cataracts, and glaucoma. But you should not wait until you "see" a problem: if you have high blood sugar, prediabetes, or diabetes, you should have your eyes examined and tested regularly (at least once a year), and sooner if you notice any change in vision.

Cataracts

A cataract is a fogging or clouding of the lens of the eye, which results in an inability to focus properly and glared or blurry vision. Although cataracts are not unique to people who have diabetes, having diabetes typically causes the disease to occur at an earlier age and to progress more rapidly than in people who do not have diabetes. Definitive treatment involves surgery.

Glaucoma

When the fluid inside the eye is unable to drain properly, pressure builds up and results in a condition called glaucoma. The pressure damages the blood vessels and nerves in the eye and causes visual problems. Primary open angle glaucoma, the most common form of glaucoma, often doesn't cause any symptoms until the disease is well advanced and there's been a significant amount of vision loss. The less common form of glaucoma, angle closure glaucoma, is usually accompanied by headache, blurred vision, watering eyes, eye pain, and seeing halos around lights.

A study of 76,000 women enrolled in the Nurses' Health

Study from 1980 to 2000 revealed that about 60 percent of all cases of primary open angle glaucoma diagnosed in the United States can be linked to patients with type 2 diabetes. Glaucoma treatment includes eye drops, laser procedures, or surgery.

Retinopathy

Diabetic retinopathy is a serious eye condition in which the blood vessels in the retina, the light-sensitive lining at the back of the eye, are damaged by glycotoxins and oxidative stress as a result of prolonged, elevated blood glucose levels. If retinopathy is not identified and treated early, it can result in blindness.

Diabetic retinopathy develops slowly over time: about 90 percent of people who have diabetes for twenty-five years or longer have blood vessel damage in their eyes. Because retinopathy takes time to develop, you have an opportunity to prevent it, including the comprehensive strategy we describe in detail in part II. All of the measures we discuss are necessary to stop the eventual loss of vision due to years of poor blood sugar control, glycation-induced damage to delicate tissues of the eye, and free-radical/oxidative stress damage. You should also have your eyes checked at least once a year (including having your pupils dilated) by an eye doctor who has expertise in diabetes-induced eye disease.

DENTAL DISEASE

Making regular dental appointments if you have prediabetes or diabetes is very important, as your chances of having dental problems increase in the presence of elevated blood glucose. The increased prevalence of dental problems, including periodontitis (bacterial destruction of the bone and tissue supporting the teeth), abscesses, gingivitis (inflamed gums), dry mouth, and soft tissue lesions, among people with prediabetes or diabetes is associated with oxidative stress, glycation-induced damage, and increased risk of infection in gum tissue. Glycotoxins damage blood vessels, collagen, and other tissues and thus compromise the health of the gums and teeth. Oxidative stress also has an important, interrelated role, as it increases the risk of infection and impairs healing of sensitive gum tissue. Long-term blood sugar elevation weakens your immune system and makes you more susceptible to infection.

Studies also show that poor dental health—the presence of periodontal infections—itself has a negative impact on the ability to control blood glucose levels. In addition, poor oral and dental health is associated with an increased risk of other diabetic complications. To help prevent periodontal disease and diabetic complications, you need to make frequent visits to your dentist (more than twice a year) for professional plaque control and scaling and to follow the recommendations outlined in the second part of this book.

ERECTILE DYSFUNCTION

Erectile dysfunction (also known as sexual dysfunction or an inability to attain and maintain an erection) affects 51.3 percent of men who have diabetes, according to a recent study completed by the Johns Hopkins Bloomberg School of Public Health. This compares with 18.4 percent of the general adult male population. The actual cause of erectile dysfunction among diabetic men is still under investigation, although several theories are being pursued. One cutting-edge idea is that a lack of nitric oxide in a region of the brain called the paraventricular nucleus triggers erectile dysfunction in men with diabetes.

Another related idea has been offered by researchers at the Brady Urological Institute at Johns Hopkins. They suggest that an abundance of a molecule called O-GlcNAc, which is present in people who have high blood sugar levels, disrupts the function of a specific enzyme (the endothelial nitric oxide synthase enzyme) that is responsible for attaining and maintaining an erection.

Low levels of the sex hormone testosterone also play a role in erectile dysfunction among men who have diabetes. One-third of men who have diabetes also have low testosterone levels. Men with diabetes should have their hormone levels checked and contemplate hormone restoration, if indicated. (See chapter 10 for a discussion of testosterone and erectile dysfunction.)

THE BOTTOM LINE

The take-home message is simple: you can prevent complications associated with diabetes, and you can greatly reduce their impact, if you minimize inflammation, oxidative stress, and glycation-induced damage from long-term blood sugar elevation and dietary glycotoxins. We describe all of those strategies in detail in the second part of this book. The tragedy of diabetic complications is not so much that they occur, but that they are having a serious, even devastating impact on people's lives when they can largely be prevented.

PART II

An Integrative Approach to Prevention and Treatment

The statistics tell a very disturbing story—metabolic dysfunction in the United States is at epidemic levels, with more than half of American adults meeting the criteria for prediabetes and another 21 million living with diabetes. Clearly, the need for effective prevention and treatment programs is more urgent than ever. The following chapters explain the details of a multifaceted, comprehensive, evidence-based approach to reverse prediabetes, prevent diabetes, or optimally manage the disease.

Our plan begins with a review of the tests we believe everyone needs to undergo to determine if they are at risk for or have prediabetes, insulin resistance, or diabetes. We'll then take an in-depth look at a cutting-edge program, which is composed of an antiglycation diet, an exercise regimen that takes minutes per day, scientifically based nutritional supplements, lifestyle modifications, and, if needed, pharmaceuticals that are integrated with the other four elements of the program. Overall, you have at your disposal a practical, comprehensive approach that is safe, easy to use, and unlike any other program you will find for prediabetes or diabetes.

Chapter 4

Looking at the Big Picture: Screening for Diabetes

It is unthinkable that in this age of advanced medical screening tests, sophisticated medical procedures, and the availability of detailed health-related information on the Internet and from other sources that the diagnosis of type 2 diabetes can be tragically delayed for as long as nine to twelve *years,* and that as many as one-third of people who have the disease are unaware that they do. Yet these statistics are true. You, your friends, and your loved ones don't want to be counted among them. You can prevent or dramatically reduce the risk of developing the complications of diabetes if you identify the ominous signs of early disease. All you need to do is undergo some simple blood tests that screen for crucial metabolic parameters, and the results will provide you and your physician with a wealth of information and a baseline from which to track any changes in your health status.

The topic of blood testing in diabetes is so important—and a bit controversial, as you will see—that we have dedicated most of this chapter to it. You will learn some surprising things, like how you and your doctor may be obtaining an incomplete picture of your metabolic health with which to monitor your condition, about what "secrets" your blood reveals, and how you and your doctor can use that information to help you prevent or dramatically reduce the risk of developing the complications of diabetes. We also take a look at a related topic: how to monitor your blood glucose levels at home.

SCREENING VERSUS TESTING

Many people use the words "screening" and "testing" interchangeably, yet these two activities are not the same. Screening is used to identify individuals who are at risk for a specific condition, while testing is used to help make a diagnosis as well as to track the progression of a disease and/or treatment. For screening to be effective, it must meet several key criteria:

1. The disease is an important health issue, and reliable tests are available.
2. The usual course of the disease is well known.
3. There are clear and undisputed benefits associated with early detection, resulting in superior outcomes when compared with delayed identification and treatment.

Diabetes emphatically meets all of these criteria, yet you may be surprised to learn that up until 2002, there were no major, randomized, controlled studies that showed just how valuable diabetes screening is at reducing the onset of overt diabetes in people at risk. That was the year the Diabetes Prevention Program trial results were published. These results highlighted the fact that intensive lifestyle modification in the areas of nutrition, exercise, and behavior—as well as the drug metformin—can *dramatically* reduce the onset of diabetes.

Briefly, the Diabetes Prevention Program Research Group assigned 3,234 nondiabetic, overweight people who had impaired fasting glucose levels to one of three groups: a lifestyle modification program with the goals of at least a 7 percent weight loss and at least 150 minutes of physical activity per week; metformin, 850 mg twice daily; or placebo pills in place of metformin. Over the three years of the study, the researchers found that, compared with placebo, lifestyle intervention reduced the incidence of developing type 2 diabetes by 58 percent and that metformin reduced it by 31 percent.

Because the prevention of diabetes is so important, this chapter focuses on how to identify if you or a loved one is at risk for insulin resistance, the key feature of type 2 diabetes. Therefore, if you have any of the symptoms or features of prediabetes and/or metabolic syndrome discussed in chapter 2, we strongly recommend that you be screened for insulin resistance. Such screening is especially critical if you are overweight, sedentary, older than forty-five, have a waist circumference of greater than 40 inches if you are a man or greater than 35 inches if you are a woman, or have a family history of diabetes, because you are at risk for diabetes.

Let's begin by looking at some simple blood tests that we believe are a great substitute for other very costly and sophisticated tests in helping to determine whether you are at risk for insulin resistance. We will then examine two more tests (hemoglobin A_{1c} and fructosamine) that are essential for checking for and following up on evidence of any glycation-induced damage to your body. We also discuss other tests that are not commonly ordered by physicians and their value in screening and testing for diabetes, including one for men only.

THE TESTS

Many people believe that undergoing a fasting plasma glucose test is all they need to do for metabolic risk assessment. We believe, however, that although this test is important and useful, fasting insulin and lipid tests are necessary screening tools for detecting insulin resistance. That being said, we recommend that all aging adults obtain yearly blood tests that provide baseline information on a variety of health parameters, including complete blood cell count, liver function tests, and serum chemistry tests. Furthermore, there are five interrelated components of metabolic health: fasting plasma glucose, fasting insulin, lipids (cholesterols and triglycerides), hemoglobin A_{1c} (Hb A_{1c}), and C-reactive protein. Once you and your doctor know your baseline values for all of these factors, you will have an accurate assessment of your current metabolic status as well as reference points for subsequent testing, which should be done regularly based on your lifestyle, current health, and individual risk factors for insulin resistance and diabetes.

Fasting Insulin Test

Many physicians do not routinely order this test, yet we believe the assessment of fasting insulin levels is an important yet simple way to help understand the risk for insulin resistance without having to undergo a more sophisticated procedure typically available only at high-powered academic research medical centers.

A quick, relatively accurate snapshot of the risk of insulin resistance can be obtained by checking a fasting insulin level at the same time as a fasting blood sugar level. If your fasting insulin and your blood glucose levels are both high, and

LOW TESTOSTERONE LEVELS IN MEN ASSOCIATED WITH TYPE 2 DIABETES AND INSULIN RESISTANCE

If you are a man who has insulin resistance and type 2 diabetes, take note. Many men in your situation have low testosterone levels. A recent study published in the *European Journal of Endocrinology* (June 2006) showed that testosterone replacement therapy in men with low testosterone levels at baseline and type 2 diabetes reduces insulin resistance and improves glycemic control. A study published a few years ago by Swedish researchers showed that testosterone restoration in middle-aged obese men was associated with significant improvements in abdominal obesity, insulin resistance, and reductions in diastolic blood pressure and cholesterol. The message? Get your testosterone levels checked.

your waist circumference is greater than 40 inches (man) or 35 inches (woman), you are at a high risk of insulin resistance.

High insulin levels (fasting hyperinsulinemia) can be defined as levels equal to or greater than 15 µU/mL (microunits per milliliter), but levels greater than 10 µU/mL also suggest risk. (Please note: in addition to insulin resistance, elevated insulin levels can indicate acromegaly, Cushing's syndrome, insulinoma, or fructose or galactose intolerance, or they may be the result of the use of prescription drugs such as levodopa, oral contraceptives, corticosteroids.)

If your blood sugar levels have been high for some time and your insulin levels that were initially high are now decreasing, this suggests that your beta cells are becoming less responsive to glucose, and you are at risk for developing beta-cell "burnout" and diabetes. Low insulin levels are a signal for many physicians to prescribe what we call old technology drugs, such as sulfonylureas (we discuss them in chapter 10), which prompt the fragile beta cells to pump out more insulin in a glucose-independent fashion. We disagree with this approach. Given that the core problems of type 2 diabetes involve beta-cell dysfunction and insulin resistance, we recommend new technology in this situation (when drugs are needed): exciting new drug therapies that improve beta-cell function in a glucose-dependent fashion, which we discuss in more detail in chapter 10.

Lipid Test

This test helps gauge your risk of metabolic syndrome, insulin resistance, and heart disease. Like the fasting plasma glucose test, you need to fast for ten to twelve hours before giving a blood sample for this test. Values identified include total cholesterol, high-density lipoprotein (HDL), low-density lipoprotein (LDL), and triglycerides.

Cholesterol is a substance that is often misunderstood and labeled as bad, when in fact cholesterol is essential for life. Cholesterol is critical for such functions as the manufacture of steroid hormones (such as estrogen, progesterone, DHEA, testosterone), the synthesis of bile acids, and the creation of cell membranes. Excess cholesterol has been associated with an increased risk of heart disease and stroke (to a lesser extent), but there is some interesting and controversial evidence that cholesterol may be associated with, but not be an actual cause of, heart disease.

Cholesterol is transported in the bloodstream by the lipoproteins HDL, LDL, and very low density lipoprotein (VLDL; not discussed here). LDL is commonly called "bad" cholesterol because elevated levels of it are associated with coronary artery disease. HDL transports excess cholesterol back to the liver for processing and is referred to as "good" cholesterol. When your lipid test results come back, here's how to interpret them.

A BETTER CHOLESTEROL TEST?

It is not unusual to see patients with type 2 diabetes who have LDL cholesterol levels that are not especially elevated. However, we know that very often in diabetics, although the "bad" LDL cholesterol level may not be very high, LDL's particle size favors the development of atherosclerosis. In fact, patients with type 2 diabetes often have small, dense LDL particles, which are much more susceptible to oxidation and the promotion of atherosclerosis (hardening of the arteries).

A potentially better cholesterol test is called the VAP (Vertical Auto Profile) test, which helps identify the size of a variety of cholesterol particles in your blood, including LDL cholesterol.

For more information on the VAP test, speak to your doctor or go to www.lef.org.

- Cholesterol: less than 200 mg/dL is considered optimal and is associated with a reduced risk of heart disease. Values greater than 240 mg/dL are associated with an increased risk of heart disease relative to someone with a level less than 200 mg/dL.
- If you have diabetes, a target LDL value of less than 100 mg/dL is suggested to reduce your risk of heart attack and stroke.
- High HDL values are associated with a reduced risk of heart disease: 60 mg/dL or greater is associated with a reduced risk of heart disease; levels around 40 mg/dL are associated with an average risk; less than 40 mg/dL suggests an increased risk. Low levels of HDL cholesterol are typically seen in patients who are insulin resistant.

- Triglyceride values greater than 130 to 150 mg/dL suggest an increased risk for insulin resistance.
- A triglyceride/HDL ratio less than 2 suggests a low risk of heart disease. The triglyceride/HDL ratio is a revealing predictor of heart disease risk that is often underutilized. The lower your triglyceride level or the higher your HDL level, the smaller your ratio will be. People who have a high ratio of triglycerides to HDL cholesterol are at high risk of insulin resistance.

The dietary and other lifestyle guidelines discussed in chapters 5 through 10 of this book can help you achieve healthy triglyceride and/or cholesterol levels.

Hemoglobin A_{1c}

The hemoglobin A_{1c} (Hb A_{1c}) test is an extremely important one; it is one of several blood tests every aging person should have. Furthermore, everyone who is prediabetic or diabetic should undergo this critical test every three to four months to help them and their doctors monitor glycation and, by extension, their current and future risk of developing diabetic complications. Although this test was developed in the late 1970s and has been around for decades, it is still much underutilized. This is unfortunate, because it provides reliable, accurate, and important information about glycation and its far-reaching consequences.

The Hb A_{1c} test is like a short-term time machine: it allows physicians to look back at the preceding three to four months and evaluate the level of glycation your body has sustained over that time period. Therefore, this test allows for a much more accurate assessment of potential damage to your body than simply focusing on blood sugar levels alone. Although blood sugar has an important impact on the level of glycation occurring in your body, it isn't the sole contributing factor. We have seen many cases where blood sugar control was reasonable, yet Hb A_{1c} remained quite elevated.

One reason the Hb A_{1c} test can offer such a broad view is that glucose sticks to such proteins as red blood cells. The Hb A_{1c} test measures the average amount of glucose in the blood over the last twelve weeks, which is the amount of time red blood cells live before they are removed from circulation. Therefore, the glucose on those cells has "stuck around" for a while and provides a more accurate picture of your accumulated glycation-induced damage over the previous three months than does the result of a fasting plasma glucose test alone.

There is a fair amount of controversy over the Hb A_{1c} test. In most laboratories, a reading of 4.0 to 5.9 percent is considered normal for healthy individuals. Some health-care professionals say that a value of 7.0 percent or lower (which roughly corresponds to an average blood glucose level of 150 mg/dL or less) is a "healthy" goal for people who have prediabetes or diabetes, while the International Diabetes Federation and American College of Endocrinology recommend a value less than 6.5 percent.

We believe that aging people, as well as people who have diabetes, should strive for an Hb A_{1c} value much lower than 6.0 percent. For longevity (remember, diabetes is a form of accelerated aging), we recommend an Hb A_{1c} level of less than 5 percent.

Because of the lack of standardized measuring techniques among laboratories, you should have all your Hb A_{1c} tests read by the same laboratory or always by labs that are standardized to the national DCCT reference method. This will not be an issue if you go to the same doctor or clinic, but if you move, change doctors, or go to a different clinic, you should ask for the name of the test-reading laboratory to ensure it is the same one that read your previous tests.

Although the Hb A$_{1c}$ test typically provides useful information, it may not always be accurate if you have had a change in diet or treatment within the preceding six weeks or if you are pregnant, because glucose and insulin levels shift frequently during those times. Results can also be inaccurate if you have anemia or sickle cell disease, or have experienced blood loss in recent weeks. In these cases, an alternative test called a fructosamine test can be done.

Fructosamine Test

Also known as a glycated serum protein or glycated albumin test, this technique has been available since the 1980s, but it is rarely used. The fructosamine test for glycation is an alternative for people who are at risk of inaccurate Hb A$_{1c}$ testing results for the reasons stated above. Similar to the Hb A$_{1c}$ test, the fructosamine test can look back and reflect your level of glycation-induced damage, but for about three weeks rather than up to twelve weeks, as is possible with the Hb A$_{1c}$ test. That's because this test measures the amount of glucose that attaches to albumin and other serum proteins, which last only about seventeen to twenty-one days in the bloodstream, and thus reflects changes that occur more quickly than those measured with the Hb A$_{1c}$ test.

Unfortunately, there is no standard reference range for the fructosamine test, which makes the practical use of this test a bit more challenging than Hb A$_{1c}$. When you get your lab results, your doctor should explain the reference range used by the specific lab. A standard reference range takes into account your age, your gender, a sample population (for example, if you are pregnant, your results will be compared with those of a pregnant population), and the testing method. Generally, your doctor will look for trends: if there is a trend from a normal to a high fructosamine level, it indicates increased glycation-induced damage, while a trend from high to normal may indicate that your treatment program is working.

Fasting Plasma Glucose Test

The fasting plasma glucose test (fasting blood sugar test) is one of the most commonly used measures of metabolic health. A blood sample is collected after a ten- to twelve-hour fast to determine the level of glucose in the blood. A fasting glucose level of up to 100 mg/dL is considered to be normal (but not optimal; 70 to 85 mg/dL is best for metabolic health); 100 to 126 mg/dL indicates impaired fasting glucose (IFG) or prediabetes; and more than 126 mg/dL indicates diabetes.

If your fasting levels are greater than 100 mg/dL and you have undergone the other tests we recommend, then your doctor can make a global assessment based on the results. A diagnosis of prediabetes or diabetes should *always* prompt an Hb A$_{1c}$ test to evaluate for glycation-induced damage to your body. If your fasting plasma glucose test result is greater than 100 mg/dL and your doctor orders an oral glucose tolerance test, we strongly recommend you ask for an Hb A$_{1c}$ test, too.

C-Reactive Protein Test

In January 2003, the Centers for Disease Control and Prevention (CDC) and the American Heart Association both endorsed the C-reactive protein (CRP) test as a screening tool for coronary artery disease. Even before their endorsement, however, my colleagues and I had been recommending this test because of the importance of inflammation as a risk factor for coronary artery disease as well as stroke and various age-related diseases. Hopefully, highlighting the importance of this test will translate into more people being screened and more heart disease being prevented.

The CRP test measures the concentration of this specific protein, which is produced by the liver when inflammation is present in the body. Because inflammation is a key factor in diabetes and its complications, including heart disease, knowing whether you have an abnormal CRP level is very important.

Average values of CRP in the population range from 1.0 to 3.0 mg/dL, but the scientific evidence indicates that these midrange, average levels are not ideal. For optimal health, CRP values need to be less than 1.0 mg/dL. For example, recent findings reported in the *New England Journal of Medicine* show that people who attain the lowest levels of CRP and LDL significantly reduce the rate of heart attack.

How to Improve Your Test Results

The good news is that you can reduce your risk of future complications by identifying health problems early on and by making lifestyle modifications and other steps as outlined in detail in the upcoming chapters. It doesn't matter whether your goal is to prevent or reverse prediabetes or metabolic syndrome or to reduce the impact of diabetic complications if you already have the disease; as you bring your test values into the healthy range, you can slow or eliminate progression of disease and disease-related complications.

MEASURING BLOOD GLUCOSE

Measuring blood glucose has never been easier; there are literally dozens of types of meters you can use at home or while traveling that allow you to easily and conveniently measure your blood glucose levels. In addition, there are several sophisticated but also easy to use monitoring devices that your doctor may recommend, should you need more detailed information than a meter can supply.

Researchers at Johns Hopkins University recently published the results of a study in the *Archives of Internal Medicine* (September 2005) showing that an Hb A$_{1c}$ level above 4.5 percent significantly increases the risk of a heart attack. Recall that so-called normal levels of Hb A$_{1c}$ range up to 5.9 percent. As you can see, "normal" does not mean *optimal*.

Whether you have prediabetes or diabetes, you should test and monitor your glucose levels based on your individual needs and goals. For patients with diabetes, this means testing levels at least four times a day—for example, before breakfast, two hours after breakfast, two hours after lunch, and in the evening. Although this may sound a bit aggressive, this approach is necessary if you want to achieve optimal blood sugar control. Achieving optimal blood sugar control is critical to reducing the risk of blindness, neuropathy, kidney failure, cardiovascular disease, and other complications of high blood sugar. If you have type 1 diabetes or you are pregnant and taking insulin, we recommend *aggressive* monitoring of blood sugar levels (see "Fasting Blood Glucose Levels Defined," page 82).

Generally, people who have type 2 diabetes and want to achieve tight glycemic control need to monitor their glucose levels very frequently. You should also increase your monitoring frequency any time you add to, or otherwise change, your treatment strategy.

FASTING BLOOD GLUCOSE LEVELS DEFINED

70–99 mg/dL: normal (we believe 70–85 mg/dL is optimal)
100–125 mg/dL: prediabetes
126 mg/dL or greater: diabetes

Source: American Diabetes Association.

Portable Home Glucose Meters

New, improved blood glucose meters are being introduced all the time, and they seem to be getting smaller, faster, and more sophisticated, requiring a smaller and smaller blood sample (and thus causing less pain) to get an accurate reading. Traditional home blood glucose testing involves pricking your fingertip with a small, sharp needle (called a lancet) and placing the resulting drop of blood onto a disposable test strip that is inserted into a portable meter. Diabetes test strips are coated with chemicals (such as dehydrogenase, glucose oxidase, or hexokinase) that react with the glucose in blood. The meter determines how much glucose is present in the sample and displays the results on the meter's screen in about ten to fifteen seconds. Portable blood glucose meters vary in size, speed of reporting, cost, amount of information they can store, and whether they can connect to personal computers. Some even come equipped with an alarm that reminds you to take your sample.

If you've ever wondered why the fingertips are the usual "sticking" collection site, it's because the blood collected there shows changes much more quickly than samples taken from other sites, such as the thigh, upper arm, forearm, or base of the thumb, and thus are more reliable. Changes occur most rapidly after exercise or eating.

Care and Calibration

To help ensure your meter is providing you with accurate readings, it's important that you keep it clean and calibrated correctly. Most meters are equipped with a program that allows you to check the calibration. We also strongly recommend that you bring your meter with you to your doctor's office so you can compare its results to the sample that is measured in the office.

The test strips are very sensitive to light, moisture, and heat and must be kept in their closed container to help prevent damage. Test strips are also specific for each meter, so always be sure the code number on your meter matches the code number on your test strips. If they do not, contact your doctor and pharmacist immediately and make sure you get the proper strips.

Continuous Glucose Monitoring System

Patients and physicians have a new tool to help them make adjustments to diabetes management plans—a continuous glucose monitoring system (CGMS). Although only a few devices have been approved as of this writing (e.g., the Medtronic MiniMed and the Guardian RT), other technologies may already or soon be on the market. The current systems measure average blood glucose for up to three days, taking up to 288 measurements every twenty-four hours.

The CGMS consists of a tiny sensing device that is implanted under the skin of the abdomen and held in place with a piece of tape. The sensor transmits its readings to a pager-sized monitor, which can be worn on a belt, and either records or displays and records the average glucose level every five minutes for up to seventy-two hours. Individuals keep a paper diary of any medications used, exercise done, and meals eaten, and also can push a button on the monitor to indicate that such actions were taken. After three days, a doctor removes the sensor and transfers the stored information into a computer, where it can be displayed in graphic form and used to make adjustments to a patient's treatment plan.

GlucoWatch

In 2001, the FDA approved a watch-like meter called a Gluco-Watch, which draws minute amounts of moisture from the skin and uses imperceptible electric currents to measure blood glucose every twenty minutes for up to twelve hours. This device is not meant to replace traditional fingertip blood glucose testing, and for good reason: the readings often are not accurate, it can irritate the skin, and it only works for twelve hours at a time. However, some people use it because they are prone to experiencing dangerously low blood sugar levels (hypoglycemia) overnight, and the GlucoWatch can be programmed to sound an alarm when it detects very low blood sugar levels.

THE BOTTOM LINE

We cannot stress enough how important it is for every aging adult to be screened for metabolic disease. Blood testing for fasting plasma glucose, lipids, insulin, CRP, testosterone (men), and Hb A_{1c} provides important information on metabolic risk. Blood testing is especially critical if you have a family history of diabetes, are overweight, have a large abdominal waist circumference, and/or have other signs or symptoms of metabolic disease. For millions of Americans, the test results will be an unwelcome surprise. However, the good news is that early detection is an opportunity to prevent complications or, if caught early enough, to reverse course.

Chapter 5

Diet Is a Four-Letter Word

Our goal in this chapter is to explain how you can eat to influence the expression of your genes and, in turn, have a positive impact on insulin resistance, beta-cell function, blood glucose levels, and glycation. Now, you may be thinking, "Here it comes, more information about counting carbohydrates and calculating my fat intake," or "I hope we're not going to be reviewing the glycemic index and glycemic load. I'm sick of trying to figure out those charts."

Actually, we're going to correct some important misconceptions about the common wisdom surrounding the glycemic index. Furthermore, we're going to share with you incredibly important information that we're almost certain you've never read or heard before. We will explore what we recognize to be the critical cause of diabetic complications—glycation—and how to employ strategies to decrease the damage done to your body by excess glycation and food-derived glycotoxins. In fact, we are going to present an easy-to-follow eating plan for life, one that is delicious, practical, devoid of fad/silly diet pseudo-science, and most important, one that helps you prevent or dramatically reduce the risk of diabetic complications. We will even show you how to painlessly and effectively lose weight.

We will also reveal for the first time why *how* you prepare your food is at least as important as *which* foods you choose to eat, as well as how to identify wise food choices and include them in your diet.

GLYCEMIC INDEX: DOES IT REALLY MATTER?

If you are totally confused and frustrated by the concept, terms, and tables associated with glycemic load and glycemic index, you are not alone. Many patients have told us over the years that these aids for choosing the "right" foods to eat to prevent, reverse, or treat diabetes are not easy to use and cause many of them to throw up their hands and give up. Indeed, what many people don't know is that these tools can be *very* misleading.

Take the glycemic index, for example. Glycemic index (GI) is a measure of how quickly a specific food will raise your blood glucose level. Basically, it is commonly believed that foods that rank high on the GI charts are considered bad, while those that rank low are considered good. But if you look at the charts, cornflakes have a high GI (86–92), while a popular chocolate and peanut candy bar has a low GI (41–43). Plain boiled carrots rank very high (about 92), while a chocolate cake with frosting ranks low (38) (see www.glycemicindex.com). Does this mean you should bypass the boiled carrots and corn- flakes and munch on candy bars and chocolate cake with frosting? Of course not! However, a strict interpretation of the GI charts suggests that is what you should do.

We also feel compelled to share with you that fructose (a

simple sugar that is found in, and added to, many foods) has a low GI rating—lower than foods that are widely known for their health benefits, including many vegetables, whole grains, and legumes/beans. Compared with glucose, which has a GI value of 100, the GI of fructose is very low at 20, while sucrose (simple table sugar) has a moderately low GI value of about 55. But what most people don't know is that *fructose is easily glycated.* This critical fact makes high levels of fructose consumption a worrisome problem for anyone who is already on the fast track toward diabetes.

Common sense tells you that choosing chocolate cake with frosting and a candy bar as the cornerstone of your nutrition plan because these two foods have a low GI ranking isn't a great idea. This extreme example points out an important fact: although the GI chart does provide some interesting information about relative blood glucose response to individual foods, it is flawed and has major limitations for use.

Many hardcore advocates of the GI may be distressed by the results of a study published in February 2006 in the *British Journal of Nutrition.* The investigators found no significant correlation between the GI of foods and the blood sugar levels of more than one thousand people who plotted their food intake for five years.

All of this information is not to say that the GI charts are useless as tools. In fact, there is scientific data to support the idea that consuming a diet very high in carbohydrates may negatively impact blood glucose levels and lipid profiles in people who have established insulin resistance or type 2 diabetes. However, the limitations of GI lists need to be noted, as many people have made them their be-all and end-all for diet and nutrition.

One limitation is that GI values do not account for the fact that most meals contain a variety of foods. For example, have you ever eaten a pound of raw carrots as a meal? Or do you

INFLUENCE OF GLYCEMIC INDEX ON GLYCEMIC RESPONSE, APPETITE, AND FOOD INTAKE IN HEALTHY ADULTS

High glycemic index (GI) diets are commonly promoted as a way to enhance appetite and promote weight gain. Support for these ideas is mainly based on the results of very short term studies done under artificial settings. So a study by Brazilian researchers published in September 2005 in the peer-reviewed journal *Diabetes Care* put these ideas to the test. Two groups of adults consumed either only low- or only high-GI foods for eight days under carefully controlled conditions. At the end of the eight days, the researchers found that there were no significant differences in plasma glucose or insulin responses, appetite ratings, or food intake between the two groups.

know anyone who eats a half pound of rice cakes for dinner? People eat meals that consist of many different food components. Deciphering the GI value of mixed meals is exceedingly complex and impractical. In addition, GI values are affected by how foods are prepared. Boiling spaghetti for twelve minutes instead of seven, for example, changes the GI value for spaghetti (the longer you boil it, the higher the GI value).

Rather than fuss with the GI charts, a far more useful way to minimize complications from diabetes is to consume a nutritionally complete diet that limits the consumption of dietary glycotoxins.

AN ANTIGLYCATION EATING PLAN

This innovative eating plan allows you to reduce a key factor involved in diabetes—glycation. Reducing food-derived glycotoxins in your diet can have a significant positive impact on your health. Our easy-to-follow eating plan, which we explain in this chapter and illustrate with a menu and recipes in the next chapter, will go a long way toward reducing the negative impact of glycation on your body.

DIETS HIGH IN GLYCOTOXINS INDUCE ENDOTHELIAL DYSFUNCTION AND INFLAMMATION IN DIABETES

A group of nonsmoking patients with diabetes were divided into two groups: one group consumed a diet high in glycotoxins, the other a diet low in glycotoxins. Results of the six-week study, published in *Proceedings of the National Academy of Sciences* in 2002, showed that patients in the high-glycotoxin group had a 35 percent increase in serum levels of C-reactive protein, an 86 percent increase in serum tumor necrosis factor-alpha levels (a marker of inflammation), and a 20 percent decrease in the level of a key marker of endothelial function. Patients in the low-glycotoxin group showed a decrease in these signs of inflammation.

The key factor in avoiding food-derived glycotoxins is temperature. Foods high in protein and fat (such as animal products like beef, pork, poultry, fish, seafood, and lamb) as well as foods high in fructose that are cooked, heated, or processed at high temperatures are loaded with glycotoxins. Overall, foods in the fat and meat (protein) groups contain thirtyfold and twelvefold higher advanced glycation end product (AGE) content, respectively, than foods in the carbohydrate group. Fresh fruits, vegetables, whole grains, raw nuts, and other unprocessed, unrefined foods have low levels of glycotoxins.

Be on the lookout for foods that are broiled, barbecued, grilled, fried, or oven roasted—these cooking methods employ high temperatures and dry cooking conditions, which generate high levels of dietary glycotoxins. High-temperature cooking methods should be used sparingly—certainly not every day and only a few times a week if possible. Instead, prepare your foods at temperatures less than 250°F to avoid the formation of dietary glycotoxins. Such methods use liquids and lower cooking temperatures and include poaching, steaming, braising, stewing, and slow cooking (as in a slow cooker).

Here's a quick comparison of the glycotoxin content of some common foods. The AGE content of beef boiled for one hour is 22 kU/g, while broiling beef for fifteen minutes results in a value of 60 kU/g. It doesn't make much difference whether you broil or fry a chicken breast for fifteen minutes; you will end up with about the same amount of AGEs: 58 kU/g and 61 kU/g, respectively. When it comes to tofu, the choice between raw (8 kU/g) and broiled (41 kU/g) is quite dramatic. At the other end of the scale are fresh fruits and vegetables, which barely make the charts (apples 0.13 kU/g, bananas 0.01 kU/g, and carrots 0.1 kU/g).

IDENTIFY THE CORNERSTONE OF YOUR PLAN

Among the questions most people ask when they talk about diet and nutrition are, "How much protein do I need?" "Should I count carbs?" "How much fat should I be eating?" Macronutrient levels (the amounts of protein, carbohydrate, and fat) in our antiglycation eating plan can be adjusted to meet your individual needs.

- Eat 15 to 25 percent of calories as protein (use the lower range if you have diabetic kidney disease, because high levels of dietary protein can stress the kidneys).
- Eat 25 to 35 percent as fat—mostly monounsaturated fats (found in relatively high amounts in olives, peanuts, sunflower seeds, and avocados) as well as adequate amounts of essential fatty acids from omega-6 and omega-3 fat sources. Since the vast majority of Americans have an imbalance of omega-6 to omega-3 fats, we recommend focusing on eating foods that contain omega-3 fats, such as walnuts, flaxseed, and fish (salmon, tuna, sardines, and mackerel are particularly rich sources of long-chain omega-3 fatty acids like DHA and EPA, which we discuss in chapter 8).
- Eat 45 to 60 percent as carbohydrates, primarily complex carbohydrates that are rich in soluble fiber. *Oatmeal Yams Brown rice Sweet Potatos Strawberries blueberries Multigrain, Wholewheat mangos, peaches & pears*

The aforementioned information is presented as a guide. There is no compelling reason for you to studiously memorize it and rigidly count carbohydrates or ponder every single macronutrient you put into your mouth. Instead, we want you to keep the above percentages in the back of your mind and then focus on adopting the recommendations in the next three guidelines. When you do, you will discover that your blood glucose levels improve, your energy increases, and unwanted pounds drop away. You won't feel hungry or deprived, especially if you follow the recommendations later in the chapter under "Lose Weight, Feel Full, Live Longer." These are just some of the things you'll notice, because behind the scenes, your diet will be having a positive impact on beta-cell function, insulin sensitivity, and the expression of genes involved in glucose metabolism.

CHOOSE GLYCOTOXIN-FREE FOODS

When we first introduced the idea of glycation in chapter 1, we noted that elevated blood sugar levels as well as the food you eat contribute to this damaging process. Food-derived glycotoxins do their damage in several ways. Those glycotoxins found in foods cooked or otherwise prepared under high heat (such as broiling, grilling, and frying) accumulate in tissues and organs throughout the body and remain there for a very long time. Although the rate of absorption of food-derived glycotoxins is not very high, the body's ability to remove (through excretion), those that are absorbed is limited. Studies show, for example, that although about 70 percent of the glycotoxins you eat escape being absorbed by the digestive tract (the body does have ways to resist these invaders), only 33 percent of the absorbed glycotoxins show up in the urine over a forty-eight-hour period. This means that the glycotoxins are deposited in tissues of the body, where they can wreak havoc.

To help you get started on your antiglycation eating program, let's look at how to choose and prepare glycotoxin-free foods.

Proteins

It makes sense to maximize the benefits you get from your food choices, so when you consider protein foods, choose items that contain not only a good amount of protein but also a healthy fat profile whenever possible. These proteins can be found in the table "Protein Sources." Include a small portion of proteins cooked with liquid at low temperatures in your diet several times a day.

PROTEIN SOURCES

- beans (adzuki, black, garbanzo, kidney, navy, pink, pinto, white)
- lentils and split peas
- soybeans and soybean-based foods (tofu, tempeh)
- seitan (wheat gluten foods; avoid if you are wheat-sensitive or have celiac disease)
- chicken and turkey (organic)
- eggs (organic)
- fish (especially cold-water fatty fish, such as salmon, tuna, and herring)
- nuts (walnuts, almonds, hazelnuts; not peanuts). Another benefit of nuts and seeds is the great amount of essential fatty acids found in these foods.
- lean, grass-fed beef (grass-fed beef provides a superior fatty acid profile). American diets by and large contain great amounts of saturated fat and omega-6 fatty acids and are relatively deficient in omega-3 fats. Grass-fed beef provides a fatty acid profile superior to corn-fed beef raised on synthetic anabolic steroids and growth-promoting agents that are used to quickly fatten and mature the cattle.
- cheese and yogurt (organic)

Carbohydrates: The Benefits of Soluble Fiber

Any mention of carbohydrates throws many people into a state of confusion: there are so-called good and bad carbs, complex carbs, high- and low-fiber carbs, sugars and starches, and so on. We will cut through the carb confusion and provide you some practical tips so you can break free of the bonds of food-restriction thinking.

Our eating plan maximizes carbohydrate sources that are rich in soluble fiber. Soluble fiber is an unsung hero in the fight against diabetes and premature aging, so we urge you to make good use of this underutilized food component. Soluble fiber includes gums, mucilage, and pectins, all of which are found primarily in plant cells. One of the most important qualities of soluble fiber is its ability to help regulate blood glucose levels: it absorbs water in the intestinal tract, combines with the digesting food to make a gel, and thus slows the rate at which glucose is metabolized and absorbed from the intestines. This slowing process also steadies the rate of insulin secretion. Another fantastic benefit of eating soluble fiber is that it can help you lose weight. It adds bulk to your diet, so it helps you feel full and more satisfied, and thus less likely to overeat. Therefore soluble fiber is an easy, inexpensive way to help curb your appetite. As a bonus, soluble fiber fills you up without adding calories. Furthermore, when you eat high-fiber foods along with foods that contain fat and cholesterol, the fiber helps to decrease the absorption of dietary fat.

But wait—there's more!

Scientific studies also show that soluble fiber reduces blood levels of cholesterol, a concern for many people with high blood sugar or diabetes, without lowering levels of the good cholesterol, HDL. Studies suggest that if you were to increase your daily intake of fiber by 10 grams (the average American adult eats a paltry 11 grams of fiber daily), you could reduce your risk of dying from heart disease by 17 to 29 percent. Fiber also helps prevent constipation, promotes the growth of healthy bacteria in your intestinal tract, and may reduce your risk of developing colon cancer. Fiber does all this and has no calories. What a bargain! Make sure you include several items from the

"Good Sources of Soluble Fiber" (page 96) at every meal. You will find some delicious ways to enjoy these carbohydrates in chapter 6.

If you are eating less than the recommended amount of fiber daily (25 to 30 grams), we recommend that you gradually add fiber-rich foods and/or soluble fiber supplements to your diet and increase your water consumption. Do not suddenly and dramatically increase your intake of fiber, or you will likely experience some bloating, gas, and other general gastrointestinal discomfort. Begin slowly by adding more soluble fiber–rich foods and/or soluble fiber supplements each day. For example, add one-half cup of beans, lentils, or split peas to your food intake daily. Or have oatmeal for breakfast several times a week and change the flavor each time: try adding flaxseeds (don't cook with flaxseeds or flax oil, because the high heat can damage their delicate essential fats), cinnamon (this spice actually offers great benefits for blood sugar regulation—more on this in chapter 8), berries, or chopped figs. Increasing the amount of fiber in your diet with foods and soluble fiber supplements until you reach your target should take several weeks or longer, depending on how quickly you adapt to the increase and what your current intake is.

Healthy Fats

There's more than one side to every story, and this holds true for the subject of dietary fat. Fat is calorie dense, and even eating the "good" fats in large amounts can add inches to your waistline. Yet your body needs a certain amount of fat, as fats are critical for the body to perform essential functions (see "Benefits of Dietary Fats," page 98). The best way to manage fats in your diet is to balance them: focus on eating the fats that are known to be beneficial (such as monounsaturated and omega-3 fats). It's important to note here that it is best to

GOOD SOURCES OF SOLUBLE FIBER

Note: We did not include the amount of soluble fiber in these foods because fiber content can vary significantly due to growing conditions and how the produce was processed or stored. The following foods are good sources of soluble fiber:

Apples	Oat bran
Apricots	Oranges
Asparagus	Parsnips
Bananas	Pears
Barley	Pinto beans
Beets	Plums
Black beans	Potatoes
Broccoli	Prunes
Brown rice	Psyllium
Brussels sprouts	Quinoa
Carrots	Rice bran
Chestnuts	Rolled oats
Collard greens	Rye
Figs	Soybeans
Garbanzo beans	Summer squash
Grapefruit	Sweet potatoes
Green peas	Tangerines
Kidney beans	White beans
Lentils	Wild rice
Lima beans	Winter squash
Mango	Yams
Navy beans	Zucchini

get more omega-3 fatty acids in your diet while also optimizing the ratio of omega-3 to omega-6 fatty acids. Americans generally consume too many omega-6 fatty acids, which are found mainly in vegetable oils. Evidence suggests that the ratio of omega-6 to omega-3 fatty acids should be no greater than 4:1, and 3:1 is even better. Most Americans have an omega-6 to omega-3 profile of 10:1 or greater. Evidence suggests that an imbalance of this type may increase the level of inflammation in the body and increase the risk of heart disease, arthritis, and certain types of cancer, including prostate cancer.

For millions of years, humans evolved on a diet rich in natural omega-3 food sources, including free-range game, fish, marine mammals, nuts, and fresh seaweed. In the early twentieth century, however, food manufacturers in the industrialized nations began literally pouring corn oil—a source of omega-6 fatty acids—into the food chain. This was accompanied by a decline in consumption of fish and wild game and a dramatic increase in the use of grains (another source of omega-6) to feed livestock. These factors, along with the popularity of fast-food restaurants and processed foods that contain vegetable oils, combined to drastically alter the balance between omega-6 and omega-3 in the Western diet.

Generally, no more than 10 percent of your calories should come from saturated and trans fat (and your goal should be to minimize the amount of trans fat in your diet as much as possible), and since people with diabetes are at high risk for or

BENEFITS OF DIETARY FATS

Essential fatty acids

- help promote healthy nerve function
- help your body absorb the fat-soluble vitamins (A, D, E, and K)
- keep your brain in good running order; your brain is composed of 60 percent fat and needs an optimal balance of omega-3 and omega-6 fatty acids to function
- help the immune system operate at its best, which is necessary for fighting infections, stimulating wound healing, and reducing the risk of cancer, among other critical tasks
- help skin, hair, and nails stay healthy and look beautiful

have heart disease, you should ideally limit these fats even further, to around 7 percent. In addition, studies suggest that the high intake of saturated fat worsens insulin resistance in obese individuals.

Since most Americans are deficient in omega-3 fatty acids and consume too much omega-6 fat, we need to focus on monounsaturated and omega-3 sources (see "Beneficial Fats," page 100). Monounsaturated fats such as olive oil have a number of beneficial effects. For example, studies show that people who consume olive oil as their main source of fat have lower rates of cardiovascular disease. Omega-3 fatty acids provide a long list of benefits; for example, they decrease risk factors for cardiovascular disease, such as high triglyceride and LDL cholesterol levels; they improve brain function and concentration, boost energy production, enhance mood, improve blood pressure, reduce cancer risk, and help reduce fat production.

The fats that you need to avoid are the following:

• trans fats, which can be identified on food ingredient lists as partially hydrogenated oil, shortening, or hard margarine. All food labels are required to state the item's trans fat content per serving, although a value of zero (0) grams per serving can mean the serving contains up to 0.4 grams (manufacturers are not required to reveal any amount less than 0.5 grams per serving). Trans fats are typically found in commercially processed foods that have been prepared under conditions of high heat, such as snack foods (for example, potato chips and roasted nuts), frozen foods (including entrées, snacks, whole dinners, desserts), commercially made cookies and crackers, packaged dinners, and baked goods

• saturated fat, found primarily in animal products (meat, poultry, whole-fat milk and dairy products, lard)

The bottom line is this: think olive oil, fish, and green leafy vegetables, and go light on meats and processed foods. You will see many food suggestions and recipes that incorporate a balance of healthy fats in chapter 6.

PREPARING AND ORDERING ANTIGLYCATION FOODS

When it comes to eating to prevent diabetes, please remember that it's not only *what* you eat that's important, it is *how* it is prepared. For example, given a choice of roasted, grilled, or steamed carrots or corn on the cob, which cooking method

BENEFICIAL FATS

Sources of Monounsaturated Fats

Avocados
Cashews
Hazelnuts
Macadamia nuts
Oils: olive, sunflower, safflower, almond, and canola
Olives
Peanuts

Sources of Omega-3

Best:	Moderate:
Atlantic salmon	Albacore tuna
Bluefin tuna	Leafy green vegetables
Flaxseed	Navy and kidney beans
Herring	Oysters
Pacific and jack mackerel	Pollock
Rainbow trout	Soybeans
Sardines	
Striped bass	
Walnuts	

SOURCE: USDA National Nutrient Database for Standard Reference, release 15.

should you select if you want to help avoid the food-derived glycotoxins that promote nerve and blood vessel damage, both of which cause and contribute to major complications of diabetes? If you guessed that steaming is better than roasting or grilling, you're right.

What's Cooking

The problem is not with the carrots or corn itself. The key issue is how the food is prepared. Processing and cooking foods at high temperatures results in what is called the Maillard reaction, in which sugars (those that are a natural part of the food or those that have been added, such as fructose and corn syrup), proteins, and some fats interact and form advanced glycation end products (AGEs) and advanced lipoxidation end products (ALEs), as discussed in chapter 1.

When you cook foods using intense heat and without water or other liquids, such as broth or wine, the sugars bind nonenzymatically to proteins (collagen and elastin fibers) and form glycotoxins. Visual evidence of this chemical reaction is the browning reaction seen in food cooked under high, dry heat. The cookies and cake in the oven, the chicken on the grill, and the potatoes in the frying pan are all browning and manufacturing AGEs and ALEs, increasing your risk of developing diabetic complications and speeding up the aging process itself. Cooking with liquids, however, inhibits the nonenzymatic attachment of sugar and fat to proteins.

"The idea that how I cook my food can have such a tremendous impact on my diabetes is just incredible to me," says Jean, a fifty-one-year-old court clerk. "I was so excited when I learned about glycation and glycotoxins, how broiling, barbecuing, and grilling are damaging my health. It was enough to make me change how I cook and what I order when I eat out, and now I feel much more in control of my diabetes and my life."

Let's consider the carrots and corn mentioned previously. Steaming them involves boiling water (212°F) for, say, five minutes, while roasting or grilling them involves very high temperatures (400°F or higher). If you have high blood glucose levels, which typically greatly accelerates the biochemical reactions that lead to glycation inside the body, eating foods that are cooked with high heat for long periods of time adds food-derived glycotoxins, which further adds fuel to the fire in terms of glycation. Cooking meats at high temperatures also creates other health hazards, such as the formation of gene-mutating toxins—carcinogens—that significantly increase your risk of cancer (see "Cook to Your Health," page 103).

Eating Out

Following an antiglycation eating plan when dining out is easy. One tip is to always verify with the waitstaff how a particular menu item is prepared. If you don't see what you want, ask if a particular item can be made for you. For example, if a fish dish on the menu is offered grilled, ask if it can be poached. Request steamed vegetables instead of roasted or grilled vegetables. Choose the poached chicken or slow-cooked beef stew entrée instead of the broiled steak or stir-fried chicken.

Here are some other tips to consider when eating out.

• Don't stop at fast-food establishments. Most items in fast-food restaurants are *loaded* with glycotoxins. Examples of foods very high in diabetes-accelerating and premature aging–promoting glycotoxins include grilled hamburgers, fried chicken, deep-fried onion rings, and French fries.

• Call ahead and ask if the restaurant's chef can prepare a specific entrée for you using low-temperature cooking methods that use liquid, like braising, poaching, and stewing.

• Be creative. If the restaurant does not have anything appropriate among the entrées, order items from the appetizer, soup, salad, and side dish sections of the menu.

• Bring your own dressing or condiments. Your freshly

made olive or flaxseed oil dressing can be the perfect topping for your restaurant salad as opposed to saturated fat–laden, glycotoxin-loaded commercial salad dressings.

• Start your meal with broth-based soup or a leafy green salad spritzed with olive oil and vinegar.

COOK TO YOUR HEALTH

DO: Marinate foods in liquids and seasonings: lemon juice, dry wine, broth, olive oil, cider vinegar. Feel free to add herbs and spices, including garlic, mustard, thyme, sage, tarragon, and others. Marinating foods can help delay the reactions that lead to glycotoxin formation.

DO: Eat foods prepared using low-heat cooking methods that employ water or liquid, like poaching, stewing, braising, boiling, steaming, slow-cooker cooking, and so on. Include a raw vegetable salad (and fruit) every day.

AVOID: broiling, frying, hot-oven roasting, grilling, barbecuing.

LOSE WEIGHT, FEEL FULL, LIVE LONGER

Feeling full or no longer feeling hungry—also known as satiety—by eating nutritious, lower-calorie foods is a very effective way to lose and manage weight. Maintaining a stable and healthy body weight is a key component of not only diabetes prevention but also diabetes management. In fact, we have observed several patients who no longer needed blood sugar–reducing pharmaceuticals after they lost a sufficient amount of weight. These cases are inspiring examples of the power of weight loss and the associated improvements in glycemic control.

Much has been written about how to lose weight, and unfortunately the majority of the information is based on misinterpreted science or pseudoscientific mumbo jumbo. Life-threatening complications can result from strictly following some of the popular diet "expert" advice. Although what we have to say here won't make us popular with the fake science crowd or sell a lot of poorly conceived diet books, the basic, unsexy truth about how to effectively lose weight is this: you need to find a way to eat fewer calories and still feel full and satisfied. The wonderful thing about this very simple approach is that it frees you from arbitrarily vilifying entire food classes (as in "carbs make you fat," "fat makes you fat") as well as worrying about eating incorrect foods for your "type," meticulously calculating precise ratios of protein/carbohydrate/fat, and doing other time-wasting activities. Our goal is to provide you with a scientifically sound yet innovative lifelong eating strategy that you can live with each and every day. Furthermore, the long-term benefits of this strategy include the prevention of metabolic disease as well as slowed aging and extended life span.

Achieving satiety is not hard to do. Basically, the more fiber, protein, and water a food item contains, the longer it will satisfy you. Stated another way, foods that have a low energy density, or relatively few calories per ounce, will make you feel full longer. Both water and fiber add bulk without piling on calories, and because they do, you can actually eat *more* food rather than less, which means you won't feel like you are depriving yourself. Fortunately, there are a great many high-fiber, water-dense foods; in fact, you will notice that many of them are also in the list of beneficial carbohydrates (see "Foods That Fill You Up," page 106). And you can do a lot of delicious, creative things with all of these foods, so you will never have to feel like you're on a diet—because you won't be! However, you should see the pounds dropping off in a gradual, steady, and sane manner.

ENERGY DENSITY AS A KEY STRATEGY FOR LONG-TERM WEIGHT LOSS

Energy density is a key feature of a long-term weight management diet. Basically, food that is higher in water and fiber content tends to be lower in energy density. For example, 1 pound of carrots weighs the same as 1 pound of butter, but the carrots are much less energy dense and lower in calories (due to the high water and fiber content) as compared to calorie-rich butter.

Research backs up the claims that consuming foods high in water and fiber content is a great long-term weight management strategy. For example, researchers at Pennsylvania State University published the results of two recent trials in the *American Journal of Clinical Nutrition* (May and June 2007). These trials showed that there were significant reductions in body weight over a six-month period associated with the highest level of water- and fiber-rich foods compared to the lowest, as well as significant advantages in terms of weight loss over one year.

For example, say you have some fresh hummus (a good source of protein and fiber) and you want to put it in a whole-wheat pita with some alfalfa sprouts or cucumber. Instead of the pita, substitute water- and fiber-rich romaine lettuce leaves. Wash two large romaine leaves, spread a thin layer of hummus on one of them, add some sprouts and thinly sliced cucumber, place the other leaf on top, and then roll up the leaves and hummus like a jelly roll. You just made a hummus sandwich that contains fewer calories and more water and fiber than a pita sandwich.

Another tip is that you can put the brakes on your hunger by

FOODS THAT FILL YOU UP

Susanna Holt, Ph.D., and her associates at the University of Sydney in Australia conducted research on satiety and developed a diet concept called the Satiety Index. This index ranks foods according to their ability to satisfy hunger, using white bread as the baseline. Foods ranked higher than white bread provide greater satiety; those ranked lower provide less. Here are some of the foods that ranked greater than 100 on the index.

Boiled potatoes—ranked the highest!	Apples
Wheat pasta	Oatmeal
Lentils	All-Bran
Baked beans	Fish
Grapes	Eggs
Oranges	Popcorn

Source: Holt, S. *Eur J Clin Nutr,* Sept. 1995; 49:675-90; Rolls, B. *Am J Clin Nutr* Jan. 2006; 83:11-17.

beginning your main meal with a small bowl of vegetable soup made with a low-sodium vegetable or chicken broth or with a leafy green salad with tomatoes, onions, cucumber, and other water-rich vegetables, along with a sprinkle of olive oil and vinegar. A moderate-size salad or broth-based soup can help you feel full faster without contributing many calories.

Here are a few more ideas on how you can reduce the energy density of your food and feel full and satisfied.

- Choose whole fruit over fruit juice—not only do you want the soluble fiber in the fruit, but commercially made fruit juices are pasteurized at high temperatures to kill bacteria. Cooking foods high in fructose (like fruit juice) is a great way to generate health-damaging dietary glycotoxins.

- When making a stew that calls for meat and vegetables, reduce the meat portion by half and substitute more water- and fiber-rich vegetables.

- When having pasta, reduce the serving by half and stir in an equal amount of steamed fiber- and water-rich vegetables.

- When making a sandwich, reduce the meat, fish, or cheese portion by half and add sliced tomato and cucumber, sprouts, lettuce, and onion to increase the water and fiber content.

- Jazz up fresh, unpasteurized fruit juice by mixing equal parts juice and seltzer. You can also freeze this mixture in ice cube trays or ice pop makers and have frozen treats.

- For a snack, choose an apple or pear instead of potato chips or pretzels, or grapes instead of raisins. Fresh fruit is much lower in calories than potato chips and also contains many fewer food-derived glycotoxins than potato chips, which are fried or baked in oil at high temperatures.

- When making egg or chicken salad, reduce the amount of the main ingredient by half, and substitute chopped celery and green pepper, shredded carrot, or radish and minced onion.

- Top your potatoes and vegetables with chopped tomatoes or salsa, or lemon juice and herbs, instead of sour cream, butter, or trans fat–laden hard margarine.

- If a broth-based soup seems too thin for you, add some pureed vegetables to the broth to make it thicker.

WHAT ABOUT SUPPLEMENTS?

A question many people ask is, "Why should I take supplements when I can get all the nutrients I need from my food?" The problem with this question is that the premise is wrong: the vast majority of people *do not* get all the nutrients they need. How many people eat a perfect diet? How many men, women, and children consume the recommended five or more servings of fresh fruits and vegetables daily, along with whole grains, raw nuts, and high-quality protein sources or consume an optimal ratio of less than 4 to 1 of omega-6 and omega-3 fatty acids daily? The unfortunate truth is that most people tend to eat too many foods that are nutritionally deficient (for example, foods that are refined, commercially processed, or overloaded with saturated fat and omega-6 fats). Another factor that robs you of the nutrients you should get from your food is that many fresh fruits, vegetables, and other unrefined foods are lower in important nutrients than they should be because of adverse growing conditions, poor food handling techniques, poor cooking methods, and poor soil quality low in trace minerals.

"The alarming fact is that foods . . . now being raised on a million acres of land that no longer contains enough of certain needed minerals, are starving us, no matter how much of them we eat." You may think this statement, voiced in the U.S. Senate, is contemporary, yet it was made in 1936. The passage of time hasn't made the fact any less true; indeed, since then, the quality of crops has grown worse. According to figures from the U.S. Department of Agriculture for the period 1963 to 1992, the vitamin and mineral content of fruits and vegetables declined dramatically: for example, calcium declined by 30 percent, iron by 32 percent, and magnesium by 21 percent in selected crops.

America is a fast-food nation. If we aren't picking it up at a drive-through window, we're nuking it in a microwave. We cook fast, eat fast, live fast, and are on the fast track for dying due to diabetes, obesity, and heart disease. Supplements are not a panacea for a nutritionally deficient diet. They are exactly what their name implies: *supplemental.* Our advice is to follow the antiglycation eating guidelines that we offer you and to supplement it with selected, scientifically tested micronutrients to best support and maintain your health.

THE BOTTOM LINE

An antiglycation eating plan, which also includes foods that help you feel full without adding lots of calories, is scientifically sound, delicious, satisfying, and one that is easy to follow for the rest of your life. Here are some key points to remember as you look ahead to the next chapter, in which we offer you some great ideas and recipes for antiglycation eating.

• There are no forbidden foods or dangerous fad-dieting rules in our program.

• Focus on making better, more intelligent food choices and using lower-temperature methods of preparation (those that use liquids and temperatures less than 250°F, which do not promote a high degree of glycotoxin formation). This can be accomplished easily if you poach, stew, slow braise with liquid (wine, water, broth), and so on, all of which help hold the cooking temperature within a better level (no more than 212°F).

• Focus on eating fresh foods and foods cooked without exposure to intense, dry heat to limit your exposure to glycotoxins. (Please note: lengthy cooking times with intense heat, such as dry-heat oven temperatures of 400°F or more, greatly increase glycotoxin formation in food.)

- Include several servings of foods rich in soluble fiber and/ or omega-3 fatty acids every day. These foods include cold-water fish, walnuts, whole flaxseed, barley, oatmeal, and yams.

- Avoid high-protein and/or high-fat animal foods prepared at high temperatures, such as grilled hamburgers and hot dogs, barbecued steak, broiled chicken, and deep-fried fish.

- Avoid or greatly limit your intake of prepackaged, preserved, pasteurized, homogenized, and refined foods, including luncheon meats and commercially prepared baked goods. All of these items have been exposed to high heat at some point during their production and contain high levels of food-derived glycotoxins.

- Avoid simple sugars exposed to high temperatures, especially commercially pasteurized fruit juices and soda/soft drinks that contain high-fructose corn syrup. These foods contain high levels of dietary glycotoxins.

Chapter 6

An Antiglycation Eating Plan

In this chapter, we bring together the information and guidelines presented in chapter 5 and show you how easy it can be to follow an antiglycation eating plan. We realize that some of the foods and cooking methods may differ from what you are used to, so we recommend that you make changes gradually. If you are used to eating lots of grilled, broiled, fried, and roasted foods or you often eat at fast-food restaurants, the changes you make will seem more dramatic than if you currently eat lots of fresh fruits and vegetables and poach or stew your entrées. If you have never steamed your fresh vegetables or poached fresh fish or chicken, now is the time to add some inexpensive cookware (such as a steamer basket and poaching pan) to your cooking utensils.

You can dramatically reduce your intake of food-derived glycotoxins if you follow the recommended cooking methods, especially when preparing foods that contain fructose and/or saturated fats and protein (such as meat, poultry, dairy, baked goods), and you reduce the amount of refined or processed foods you eat. Do not chastise yourself if you eat French fries on occasion or indulge in barbecued chicken once in a while. The goal isn't to rigidly restrict high-glycotoxin foods but rather to adopt an eating strategy that emphasizes good food choices and safer food cooking methods for a lifetime.

You and your family can enjoy easy, delicious, and healthful foods that you can prepare yourself and that will help reduce the amount of food-derived glycotoxins you are ingesting every day. You can save the grilled burgers and French fries, the fried chicken and oven-roasted potatoes, for example, for an occasional meal. All this is possible if you follow the tips and guidelines in chapter 5 and use the menu and recipes offered in this chapter as a starting point for an easy-to-follow eating plan that will last you the rest of your life. Recipes are provided for items followed by asterisks.

FIVE-DAY MENU AND RECIPES

— *DAY 1 Breakfast* —

Breakfast Oatmeal* with 1 tablespoon ground flaxseed
½ grapefruit
Green tea

— *DAY 1 Lunch* —

Speedy Chili*
Raw vegetables (carrot sticks, cucumber slices, red pepper strips, jicama sticks) with Hummus*
Tea

— DAY 1 Dinner —

Green salad (mixed greens [arugula, romaine, spinach]) with cucumber, shredded carrot, onion, and Mediterranean Dressing*
Pasta with Mushrooms and Lentils*
Berry Mousse*
Iced or hot coffee

Day 1 Recipes

BREAKFAST OATMEAL
Serves 1

1 cup cold water
½ cup old-fashioned oats
½ teaspoon cinnamon
1 tablespoon ground flaxseed

Combine water and oats in saucepan and bring to a boil. Allow to boil on low for 3 to 5 minutes or until desired consistency. Place in bowl, stir in cinnamon, and top with flaxseed.

SPEEDY CHILI
Serves 6

1 cup water
1 medium onion, chopped
2 cloves garlic, minced
1 small bell pepper, diced
½ cup fresh tomatoes, crushed
2 cups cooked black beans
4 ounces diced green chilies
1 teaspoon ground cumin

Heat ½ cup water in a skillet and add onion, garlic, and bell pepper. Cook over high heat, stirring often, for 5 minutes. Add the tomatoes, beans, remaining water, chilies, and cumin. Simmer for about 10 to 15 minutes.

HUMMUS

Makes about 2 cups

1½ cups cooked garbanzo beans
¼ cup lemon juice
2 tablespoons raw tahini
3 green onions, chopped
1 tablespoon chopped garlic
1 teaspoon ground cumin
½ teaspoon black pepper

Place all the ingredients into a blender or food processor and process until smooth. Add a few drops of water if you want a smoother consistency.

PASTA WITH MUSHROOMS AND LENTILS

Serves 4–5

1 pound whole-wheat pasta
1½ cups low-sodium, low-fat pasta sauce
1 cup cooked lentils
1 cup sliced mushrooms
½ cup low-salt vegetable broth
Garlic powder and/or black pepper, to taste

Cook the pasta according to package directions. While the pasta cooks, combine the sauce, lentils, mushrooms, and broth in a saucepan and heat on low. Season as desired. Drain the pasta and top with the sauce.

MEDITERRANEAN DRESSING

4 tablespoons apple cider vinegar
4 tablespoons extra virgin olive oil or flaxseed oil
6 tablespoons water
20 almonds
4 teaspoons ground flaxseed
2 teaspoons sea salt
Crushed black pepper, basil, and thyme, to taste

Place all ingredients except the pepper, basil, and thyme into a blender or food processor and process until smooth. Stir in the herbs.

BERRY MOUSSE

Serves 4

1 package (about 12 ounces) low-fat, extra-firm silken tofu, crumbled
2¾ cups thawed frozen unsweetened berries, your choice
2 tablespoons agave nectar
1 tablespoon berry liqueur (optional)

Place all the ingredients into a blender and blend until smooth. Spoon into pudding dishes and refrigerate until chilled.

DISPELLING THE FLAK ABOUT FLAXSEED AND FLAXSEED OIL

- Flaxseeds can be purchased already ground or whole. Whole flaxseeds are typically available in the bulk section of the grocery store and have a longer shelf life than ground seeds. If buying whole flaxseeds, make sure there is no evidence of moisture at the point of purchase, and store them in an airtight container. Refrigerate them once you get them home.
- Grinding flaxseeds in a seed or coffee bean grinder boosts their digestibility and nutritional value.
- When buying ground flaxseeds, look for vacuum-sealed and/or refrigerated packages, as the seeds are much more susceptible to oxidation once they are ground. Store ground seeds in an airtight container and refrigerate.
- Flaxseeds can be sprinkled on cereal and vegetables, added to breakfast shakes, or mixed into muffin, bread, or cookie recipes.
- When adding ground flaxseeds to a cooked dish, do so at the end of the cooking time. The soluble fiber in the seeds can cause the liquids in the dish to thicken, and high heat damages the delicate essential fatty acids in flax (and heating/frying with flax oil under high temperature generates cancer-promoting compounds).
- Add flaxseeds to your diet gradually; use 1 teaspoon on your cereal the first few times rather than 2 tablespoons.
- Never use flaxseed oil in high-heat cooking. Add it to foods after they have been prepared.

— *DAY 2 Breakfast* —

Whole wheat cereal topped with chopped walnuts
Low-fat milk or soy beverage for cereal
Orange or berries
Green tea

— *DAY 2 Lunch* —

Red Lentil Soup*
Organic rye crackers
Iced herbal tea

— *DAY 2 Dinner* —

Poached Fish*
Yam It Up*
Steamed broccoli or cauliflower drizzled with flaxseed oil
Iced coffee or tea

Day 2 Recipes

RED LENTIL SOUP

Serves 6

7 cups water
2½ cups dry red lentils
1 large onion, minced
1 teaspoon turmeric
Pinch cayenne pepper
2–4 tablespoons fresh lemon juice
1 teaspoon ground cumin
Salt and pepper, to taste

NUTS ABOUT NUTS

When researchers compared a dietary plan that contained walnuts against two other dietary plans that didn't, they found that the men and women with type 2 diabetes who ate 30 grams of walnuts (about eight to ten nuts) daily had a significantly greater increase in their HDL cholesterol to total cholesterol ratio and in their HDL levels, and a significant reduction in their LDL cholesterol, all positive indicators for cardiovascular and overall health.

Harvard researchers also unshelled the importance of nuts in type 2 diabetes. They looked at the dietary habits of more than 83,000 women from the Nurses' Health Study over sixteen years and found that women who reported eating 1 ounce of nuts at least five times per week reduced their risk of type 2 diabetes by nearly 30 percent compared with women who never or rarely ate nuts. Risk was reduced by 16 percent in women who ate 1 to 4 ounces of nuts per week and by 8 percent among those who ate less than 1 ounce per week. Experts believe that the healthy fats in nuts allow the body to use insulin more efficiently and help regulate blood glucose levels. Women who frequently ate peanut butter (although peanuts are technically a legume, not a nut) reduced their risk of type 2 diabetes by nearly 20 percent compared with women who rarely ate peanut butter.

Combine water, lentils, onion, turmeric, and cayenne in a large pot and bring to a boil. Reduce heat, partially cover, and simmer for about 30 to 45 minutes. Stir in lemon juice, cumin, salt, and pepper.

POACHED FISH

Serves 4

½ cup dry white wine
½ cup water
1 cup fresh mushrooms, sliced
1 teaspoon dried rosemary, crushed
½ cup celery, sliced thin
1 clove garlic, chopped
½ cup carrots, sliced thin
1 cup vegetable broth
1 pound fresh salmon or halibut steaks

In a skillet, combine all ingredients except the fish. Bring to a boil, reduce heat and simmer, covered, for 5 minutes. Add the fish, and spoon poaching liquid over it. Simmer, covered, until the fish flakes easily when tested with a fork. This should take 6 to 8 minutes. Use a slotted spoon to transfer fish and vegetables to a serving dish. Keep warm while boiling the poaching liquid, uncovered, for about 5 minutes or until it is reduced to about 1/3 cup. Pour on top of the fish and vegetables.

YAM IT UP

Serves 4

2 small yams, cut into bite-size pieces
1 onion, quartered and sliced
2 garlic cloves, minced
1 tablespoon Worcestershire sauce
½ teaspoon chili paste
2 small heads bok choy, sliced thin
Juice of ½ lemon

Place the yams in a skillet and cover with water. Boil the yams, covered, for 5 to 10 minutes, or until soft. Add onion and garlic and simmer until half the water has boiled away. Add Worcestershire sauce, chili paste, and bok choy and simmer until bok choy is soft. Sprinkle with lemon juice and serve.

— DAY 3 Breakfast —

Green Omelet*
Dried figs
Coffee or green tea

— DAY 3 Lunch —

Fiesta Bean Salad*
Albacore tuna (in water) with tomato and lettuce
Iced coffee

— DAY 3 Dinner —

Vegetable Soup*
Slow-Cooked Chicken and Olives*
Squash Buckler*
Herbal tea

Day 3 Recipes

GREEN OMELET

Serves 1

½ cup spinach, chopped
½ cup mushrooms, sliced
1 egg plus 2 egg whites
2 tablespoons low-fat milk

½ cup tomatoes, chopped
3 tablespoons skim mozzarella cheese

Steam the spinach and mushrooms. In a bowl, combine the eggs with the milk. Pour into a skillet that has been sprayed with olive oil. As the omelet cooks, place the spinach, mushrooms, tomatoes, and mozzarella in the center. Fold the omelet in half and cook for 30 to 60 seconds.

FIESTA BEAN SALAD

Serves 4–6

1 cup cooked black beans
1 cup cooked pinto beans
1 cup cooked garbanzo beans
1 cup frozen corn, thawed
1 small onion, chopped
1 small red or green pepper, seeded and chopped
¼ cup olive or flaxseed oil
¼ cup red wine vinegar
½ teaspoon salt
¼ teaspoon garlic powder

Combine all ingredients and mix well. Chill.

VEGETABLE SOUP

Serves 4

3–4 tablespoons water
4 cloves garlic, minced
5 cups low-sodium vegetable broth
2 sprigs thyme

2 cups fresh spinach, chopped
1 cup red bell pepper, thinly sliced
½ cup frozen green peas, thawed
¼ cup carrots, shredded
½ cup frozen cut corn, thawed
1 cup fresh asparagus, cut

Steam/sauté the garlic in water in a heavy skillet for 1 minute. Add the broth and thyme and bring to a boil. Cover, reduce heat, and simmer for 10 minutes. Add the spinach, pepper, peas, carrots, and corn; cover and simmer for 5 minutes. Add the asparagus, cover and simmer 2 to 4 minutes, or until tender.

SLOW-COOKED CHICKEN AND OLIVES

Serves 4

4 boneless, skinless chicken breasts
½ cup red or white wine
¼ cup olive oil
1 tablespoon oregano
2 bay leaves
6 cloves garlic, crushed
1 teaspoon ground black pepper
1 teaspoon salt
2 tablespoons capers
¼ cup green olives
¼ cup black olives

Place chicken in the slow cooker. Combine the remaining ingredients and pour over the chicken. Cook on low for 6 to 7 hours.

SQUASH BUCKLER

Serves 4

¼ cup vegetable broth
½ cup onion, chopped
2 teaspoons jalapeño pepper, minced
2 cloves garlic, minced
1 cup yellow squash, sliced
1 cup zucchini, sliced
½ cup fresh corn kernels
1½ cups cooked pinto beans
1 cup fresh tomatoes (keep the juice), diced
2 cups cooked brown rice

Place the broth in a skillet over medium-high heat. Add the onion, jalapeño, and garlic and sauté for 2 minutes. Add the squash and zucchini and cook another 2 minutes. Add the corn, beans, tomatoes, and liquid. Cover, reduce heat, and simmer 8 to 10 minutes. Serve over rice.

— DAY 4 Breakfast —

Banana Oat Smoothie*
Slice organic rye bread with all-natural peanut butter
Herbal tea

— DAY 4 Lunch —

Mushroom Barley Soup*
Raw vegetables with Low-Fat Guacamole*
Iced or hot coffee or tea

— DAY 4 Dinner —

Spinach salad with shredded carrot, mushrooms, walnuts, and Mediterranean Dressing* (page 115)
Seitan Stew*
Frozen Watermelon Delight*
Green tea

Day 4 Recipes

BANANA OAT SMOOTHIE

Makes 3 cups

2 medium bananas
2 cups low-fat, fortified vanilla soy milk
½ cup quick-cooking rolled oats
2 teaspoons vanilla extract
6 ice cubes

Place all ingredients into a blender and process until smooth.

MUSHROOM BARLEY SOUP

Serves 3

2 cups plain rice milk
2 tablespoons barley flour
1 cup cooked barley
½ cup mushrooms, sliced
¼ teaspoon garlic powder
¼ teaspoon salt
Pinch each: dried marjoram, sage, thyme, dill weed

Place the rice milk and flour into a blender and process on high for a few seconds. Add the barley and blend on high

An Antiglycation Eating Plan 125

for 10 seconds. Add mushrooms, and blend just enough to coarsely chop the mushrooms. Transfer the blended mixture into a saucepan, and add all the remaining ingredients. Simmer for about 5 minutes, or until the soup has thickened.

LOW-FAT GUACAMOLE

Makes 2½ cups

1 cup fresh or frozen green peas
1 ripe avocado, peeled
½ cup fresh tomatoes, finely chopped
1 garlic clove, finely chopped
1 green onion, chopped
½ teaspoon chili powder
½ teaspoon ground cumin
Juice of 1 lemon
1 tablespoon chopped fresh cilantro
Salt and black pepper, to taste

Blanch the peas in boiling water for 2 to 3 minutes, then let them cool. Cut the avocado into large chunks. Mash the avocado and peas together with a fork or masher. If you want a very creamy consistency, use a food processor. Add the tomatoes, garlic, onion, chili powder, cumin, lemon juice, and cilantro. Season with salt and pepper if desired.

SEITAN STEW

Serves 4

1 large onion, chopped
2 carrots, diced
3 small turnips, peeled and cut into quarters

3 small yams, cut in half
½ pound mushrooms, halved
3 dried tomatoes, powdered
1 cup vegetable broth
1 tablespoon olive oil
8 ounces seitan, cut into chunks
1 teaspoon each: dried rosemary, dried thyme, dried sage
1 tablespoon miso
1–2 tablespoons arrowroot
¼ cup water
Salt and pepper, to taste

Steam the onion, carrots, turnips, and yams until the vegetables begin to soften. Transfer the vegetables to a skillet. Add the mushrooms, tomato powder, ½ cup of the broth, and the oil. Simmer for 5 minutes. Then add the seitan, dried herbs, miso, and remaining broth. Cook for about 10 minutes, or until vegetables are tender. In a cup, combine the water and arrowroot and mix well. Add to the skillet, and stir until thickened. Season as desired.

FROZEN WATERMELON DELIGHT

Serves 2

1¾ cups ice cubes
1 cup seedless watermelon, coarsely chopped
1 cup lemon-flavored herbal tea at room temperature

Place all ingredients into a blender and process on high until smooth.

— DAY 5 Breakfast —

Quinoa Breakfast*

Sliced hard-boiled egg
Green tea

— DAY 5 Lunch —

Curried Sardines*
Modified Waldorf Salad*
Herbal tea

— DAY 5 Dinner —

Split Pea Soup*
Cilantro Chicken* with brown rice
Vegetable juice with lemon

Day 5 Recipes

QUINOA BREAKFAST

Serves 2

1 cup quinoa
2 cups water
2 dates, chopped
¼ cup berries (your choice)
1 teaspoon honey
1 teaspoon cinnamon

Wash the quinoa to remove the seed cover. Bring the water to a boil and stir in the quinoa. Cover and reduce heat to low, and simmer for 15 minutes. While the quinoa is simmering, chop the dates and combine with the berries, honey, and cinnamon. Add this fruit mixture to the simmering quinoa during the last 5 minutes it is cooking.

CURRIED SARDINES

Serves 2

1 tablespoon olive oil
½ cup green pepper, chopped
1 small onion, sliced
1 cup mushrooms, sliced
1 small zucchini, sliced
1 cup fresh tomatoes, chopped
2 cans sardines
Curry powder to taste

Place oil, pepper, onion, mushrooms, zucchini, and tomatoes in a skillet and simmer on low for 3 to 4 minutes, stirring often. Add the sardines, and simmer for 6 to 10 minutes. Season with curry powder. Serve with brown rice.

MODIFIED WALDORF SALAD

Serves 2

¼ cup low-fat plain yogurt
¼ teaspoon vanilla extract
½ teaspoon salt
¼ teaspoon black pepper
1 tablespoon lemon juice
1 red apple, cubed
½ cup celery, diced
½ cup grapes, halved
¼ cup raisins
½ cup chopped walnuts
Lettuce

In a small bowl, mix together the yogurt, vanilla, salt, pepper, and lemon juice. Add the remaining ingredients except for the lettuce. Mix well and serve on lettuce leaves.

SPLIT PEA SOUP

Serves 8

2 cups dry split peas
6 cups hot water
1 cup carrots, chopped
1 cup celery, sliced
1 medium onion, chopped
2 garlic cloves, minced
½ teaspoon each: dried marjoram, dried basil
¼ teaspoon each: ground cumin, black pepper
1 teaspoon salt

Place all ingredients in a slow cooker. Cover and cook on high for 3 to 4 hours, or until split peas are soft. Or, place all ingredients in a large pot, bring to a simmer, and then cover loosely. Cook until split peas are tender, 1 to 2 hours.

CILANTRO CHICKEN

Serves 4

1 pound boneless, skinless chicken breasts
1 large lime
1 cup white wine
2 tablespoons olive oil
1 green or red bell pepper, chopped
2 small onions, chopped
1 one-inch piece of fresh ginger, peeled and sliced thin

2 tablespoons fresh cilantro, chopped
2 tablespoons reduced-sodium soy sauce
Brown rice (optional)

Cut each chicken breast into eight pieces. Cut the lime in half and peel one half. Juice the lime and set aside 2 tablespoons of juice. In a poaching pan, add the white wine and bring to a simmer. Drizzle the oil into the pan and add the chicken, pepper, onions, and ginger and cover the pan. Poach for about 5 minutes, or until the chicken is no longer pink in the center. Add the lime peel, juice, chopped cilantro, and soy sauce and stir until well mixed. Serve with brown rice.

THE BOTTOM LINE

The ideas and recipes in this chapter are only a very small sample of the delicious, healthful foods you can enjoy as part of an antiglycation eating plan. We know many people who have made the adjustments, and they have improved blood glucose and lipid levels to show for it, plus the unseen benefits of helping prevent the complications of glycation. An antiglycation eating plan is one that everyone can follow, including your partner and children.

Chapter 7

Everyone Has Twelve Minutes

When we see a patient whose glucose level is consistently high, one of the first questions we ask is, "Do you exercise?" An all-too-common response to the inquiry is "I don't have time." Exercise is a very important way to improve glucose metabolism and insulin sensitivity. And for most people, the biggest barrier to reaping the significant benefits of exercise is time.

Well, we have a solution. In this chapter, we introduce an exercise program that can completely eliminate the "I don't have time to exercise" issue.

This chapter outlines a bare-bones exercise session that burns a grand total of twelve minutes of time. The approach is a simple, scientifically validated one, yet it has been essentially overlooked by most health-care advocates when they talk about exercise and metabolic health.

The core component of our approach was born from a program originally developed for elite athletes, but you certainly don't need to be an athlete to derive benefit from the program. In fact, the approach can be adjusted to meet the needs and fitness level of anyone, from elite athlete to out-of-shape couch potato.

If you have a little more time to exercise or if you would like a change of pace, we also discuss other types of physical activities that are beneficial for improving insulin sensitivity and blood glucose control and how and when to monitor your blood glucose around your exercise sessions.

PHYSICAL ACTIVITY AND DIABETES

Physical activity has far-reaching effects and benefits for everyone. This is especially true for people who want to prevent, reverse, or better manage metabolic disease.

Effect on Blood Glucose and Insulin

One reason regular physical activity is so critical is that when you exercise, you help reverse insulin resistance at the cellular level and improve the ability of your cells to take in glucose, which in turn improves your overall glycemic control. That's why regular exercise can reverse and prevent diabetes and why it can reduce the need for medication—both antidiabetes drugs and insulin—among people who already have diabetes.

The relationship between exercise and blood glucose is clear: muscles need energy to move, and glucose is a major source of fuel that makes movement possible.

Muscles use three different types of fuel for energy: high-energy phosphates, glucose (the storage form of glucose is known as glycogen), and free fatty acids. Depending on the intensity and duration of exercise, your muscles use different fuel mixtures. For example, if you lift a very heavy weight over your head, you are primarily tapping into the phosphate system. If you decide to run 5 miles at a brisk pace, you will mainly use glycogen, while walking slowly primarily uses free fatty acids (and some glycogen as well, but not very much).

To best improve insulin sensitivity and glucose uptake by muscle cells, you should focus on exercise that stresses the glycogen system.

Effect on Metabolic Syndrome

Physical activity has an impact on the other factors that are part of insulin resistance—blood pressure, triglyceride levels, and HDL cholesterol levels. Many studies have shown that regular physical activity improves blood pressure, reduces LDL cholesterol levels, raises HDL cholesterol levels, and lowers triglyceride levels. All of these improvements are helpful in reducing the risk of heart disease.

Physical activity can also help you to maintain weight loss and lose weight when combined with a reduction in calorie intake. If you are trying to lose weight, dieting alone without regular exercise can cause you to lose lean muscle tissue, so this approach to weight loss is not optimal. Regular exercise is an important part of a long-term weight-control strategy.

Another benefit of physical activity is its ability to relieve stress and tension. This is an important though often overlooked benefit of regular physical exercise. Stress can negatively affect blood glucose levels both directly and indirectly and can have a significant effect on blood pressure. Studies show that mental and emotional stress causes blood glucose levels to rise in people who have type 2 diabetes and can cause glucose levels to rise or fall in people who have type 1 diabetes.

Georgia, a forty-nine-year-old marketing manager with type 2 diabetes, noticed that she was having an increasingly hard time keeping her glucose levels in a healthy range with diet and her oral medication. The trouble all began, she said, when she took on a major project at work that required her to take work home with her every night.

"The stress was getting to me," she says, "and it was most evident in my blood sugar levels. Even though my eating habits hadn't changed—I'm very careful about my diet—my postmeal blood sugar levels were too high. I couldn't stop working on the project, and I didn't want to increase my meds. The missing element, I decided, was exercise." Georgia began to take a brisk walk every night after work, and the results were almost immediate. "My glucose levels came down immediately," she says, "but there were other benefits, too. I felt more energized, I was able to concentrate better, and I felt much less tension in my shoulders and neck when I was working. I started with a fifteen-minute walk, and then built up to a thirty-minute walk. Once the project was over, I kept on walking! It really helps keep my blood sugar levels in line, and I feel more relaxed."

Stress indirectly impacts blood glucose levels simply because people under stress often do not take care of themselves properly. Patients often say, "I work through lunch," or "I'm too busy to check my glucose levels," or "I don't have time to eat right." Stress management skills, as we discuss in chapter 9, can help turn these health-damaging behaviors around.

Before You Get Started

Before you incorporate a new physical activity program into your life, you should talk to your doctor, have your medical history reviewed, and be examined for any signs or symptoms of heart or blood vessel disease or conditions that affect your eyes, kidneys, nervous system, or feet. Depending on your doctor's findings and your current state of health, he or she may order an exercise stress test or other tests to identify your ability to exercise or, most likely, will give you some guidelines so you can begin to get physically active right away.

Such examinations and tests by your doctor are especially critical if you already have diabetes and/or you have other medical conditions that can impact your safety when exercising. If you have some peripheral neuropathy (loss of sensation in your feet), for example, your podiatrist may recommend a specific type of athletic shoe or shoe insert and encourage you to examine your feet before and after each physical activity session. If you have high blood pressure, your doctor may advise you to avoid activities that involve straining (e.g., lifting heavy weights overhead or moving heavy furniture).

Several large studies have been conducted at the University of Georgia, one of which analyzed seventy controlled, randomized trials that included 6,807 volunteers. The investigators found that in more than 90 percent of the studies, formerly sedentary people who stayed with a regular exercise routine, including those who had medical conditions such as diabetes, experienced an improvement in fatigue compared to people who did not exercise.

Regular physical activity is very good for you—physically, emotionally, mentally—and *deep down* you know it.

Less Is More: Fitness Training the Tabata Way

What good is a recommended physical activity program if people can't or won't do it? No good at all. But there is plenty of evidence to support our exercise approach, which allows you to achieve cardiorespiratory fitness (and reduce the risk of insulin resistance and metabolic disease, and better manage diabetes) without the need to spend extensive hours in the gym exercising. Enter the Tabata protocol, a program originally developed to maximize the aerobic and anaerobic conditioning of elite athletes in the shortest time possible.

This innovative approach is named after Izumi Tabata, Ph.D., a former researcher at Tokyo's National Institute of

Health and Nutrition, who helped develop an optimal method of interval training with the head coach of the Japanese speed-skating team. The routine improves your maximum aerobic capacity, which is a measure of the maximal level at which your body is able to take in oxygen and pump oxygenated blood to muscle tissues. The Tabata approach also (simultaneously) improves anaerobic capacity, which is a measure of how effective your muscles' metabolic machinery is at working without oxygen during intense effort.

Since the Tabata protocol was originally developed as a form of interval training with world-class athletes in mind, a natural question to ask is whether this method is appropriate for or applicable to everyone. Yes, in its pure form the Tabata protocol is *really* very strenuous. However, the modified form that we recommend adjusts the approach to retain the essential structure of the exercise program while tailoring the intensity to safely fit your abilities and still get effective results.

One advantage of a modified Tabata approach to interval training is that you can use it with many different aerobic activities, including running, biking, swimming, rowing, water aerobics, elliptical training, or using a step machine. You can also alternate your activities: use a stationary bike one day, use an elliptical trainer the second day, swim the third day, and so on.

The entire modified Tabata training session, including warm-up and cooldown, takes just twelve minutes. Here's how you do it.

• Four minutes of warm-up using dynamic stretching and joint mobility movements. You can use the dynamic stretching and joint mobility exercise suggestions offered in this chapter or others approved by your doctor or physical therapist.

• Eight thirty-second intervals, each consisting of twenty seconds of (for you) relatively hard physical effort, followed by ten seconds of active rest. This thirty-second cycle is repeated seven times, for a total of eight cycles. The eight cycles take just four minutes. It is important for you to remember that the interval portion of the program is very flexible: the intensity of the effort is up to you. The harder you work during the twenty-second work periods, the greater the benefit. However, we urge you *to gradually and slowly* increase the intensity level, especially if you have not exercised in a long time. A gradual, persistent increase in exercise intensity is the way to go.

• Four minutes of cooldown using dynamic stretching and/or static stretching.

That's it! You've just completed your combined aerobic and anaerobic conditioning program for the entire day, with flexibility and joint mobility training as well. We recommend you do this routine every other day, at least three times and preferably four times per week. This program will work even better if you incorporate some strength training, which we explain in this chapter as well. Naturally, you can extend your modified Tabata program/interval-training workout by adding a few minutes to the exercise time. Some patients obtain better results by extending their cooldown sessions when they have extra time by adding a ten-minute brisk walk after they stretch at the end of the workout. The important thing is that you can make adjustments to your activity level based on your specific needs—whether you are trying to prevent diabetes, improve insulin sensitivity, reduce signs of metabolic dysfunction (e.g., high blood pressure, central/abdominal obesity), or better manage your blood sugar levels as a diabetic.

GETTING STARTED WITH A MODIFIED TABATA PROTOCOL

- Discuss your exercise plans with your doctor before you start any type of physical activity program. This is important for everyone, but especially if you have not exercised for some time, are overweight, are elderly, and/or have a history of heart disease, stroke, hypertension, respiratory problems, joint replacement, or osteoporosis.

- Select warm-up exercises from the dynamic stretching and joint mobility categories and cooldown exercises from the section in this chapter, and add in static stretching at the end of the workout. Both warm-up and cooldown exercises are *important*; do not skip them.

- Choose an aerobic activity that interests you. You don't need to do the same activity at each session—variety helps keep exercise more interesting and engages different muscles.

- Do your training sessions (with warm-up and cooldown) at least four times per week in the beginning. You can alternate the activities you perform in each of the four-minute segments to help keep it interesting.

- Keep track of your time. If you are indoors, it's helpful to have a clock with a sweeping second hand that you can watch as you work out. If you are outdoors or in a pool, you will have to count to yourself. Practice counting while watching a second hand so you can become accustomed to the rhythm.

- Begin slowly and gradually over a one- to six-week period, depending on your current state of health and fitness. You will *gradually* increase the intensity of each twenty-second period of intense physical effort over time to reach the level that's right for you. Your doctor can help guide you on how to begin.
- If you are using this method to speed up weight loss, we recommend building up to your maximum exercise effort over a six-week period and performing the exercise sessions daily.

STRENGTH TRAINING

Strength (resistance) training has typically taken a backseat to aerobic exercise and has not been emphasized as a way to improve metabolic function. This is regrettable, because for many people, long duration/low intensity aerobic workouts are just plain *boring*! Resistance exercise/strength training has marvelous, often-overlooked benefits for improving metabolic function and blood sugar control.

For example, in a study published in the *International Journal of Sports Medicine* in 1997, people with type 2 diabetes who completed a three-month strength-training program using weights two days per week experienced a significant improvement in blood glucose control and an increase in muscle mass. By improving glycemic control and reducing the potential for glycation, such training also decreases the risk of developing diabetic complications. In another study published in 1998 in *Diabetes Care*, people with type 2 diabetes were divided into two groups. One group participated in strength training, and the other was sedentary. During the four- to six-week study, people in the exercise group trained five times per week using weights that worked both the upper and lower body muscles. The study results showed that moderate-intensity training improved insulin sensitivity by an impressive 48 percent.

Strength training can literally *reverse* the aging of skeletal muscles. A study published in 2007 by the Buck Institute of Age Research compared muscle biopsies from healthy older and younger adults before and after a six-month strength-training program. Before training began, the older adults were 59 percent weaker than their younger counterparts, but after training, the difference was only 38 percent. One remarkable finding was that strength training had a direct impact on gene expression by partially reducing its negative impact skeletal muscle weakness and impairment associated with aging.

Strength-Training Guidelines

A basic strength-training recommendation from the American Diabetes Association and the American College of Sports Medicine follows:

- Participate in strength training at least two times per week.
- Do eight to twelve repetitions per set.
- Do one to two sets per exercise.
- Include eight to ten exercises in each session that target major muscle groups.

Before you get started, here are some basic guidelines to ensure your sessions are effective, safe, and fun.

- Talk to your doctor before starting strength training. This is especially critical if you have high blood pressure or any type of heart or blood vessel disease.

- Always warm up before doing strength training. Five to seven minutes of dynamic stretching and brisk walking can warm up your muscles. A five-minute cooldown that includes various stretching exercises is also recommended.

• You don't need to go to a fancy fitness club to do strength training: the proper use of free weights and/or a home gym is sufficient. It is important, however, that you have guidance on how to do strength training at home before you begin. A physical therapist or qualified fitness expert at a local health club can be helpful. You may consider taking a class on strength training offered by a local health club, community center, or hospital.

• You can do your strength training on the days you are not doing an aerobic workout or after an aerobic workout session. See which way works best for you.

• Avoid doing any movements that cause a sharp pain. It's okay to feel a "burn" in your muscles, but it's not okay to feel pain in any joint.

Strength training compares favorably with aerobic endurance training. In a four-month randomized controlled trial conducted in Vienna, Austria, the type 2 diabetics who participated in the strength-training portion of the study enjoyed an impressive improvement in Hb A_{1c} (from 8.3 percent to 7.1 percent), as well as significant reductions in blood glucose, insulin resistance, total cholesterol, and triglyceride levels and a beneficial increase in high-density lipoprotein (HDL). The diabetics in the traditional low-intensity endurance-training segment of the trial, however, did not experience significant beneficial changes.

Dynamic Versus Static Stretching: It Makes a Difference

You've been told for years that it's best to stretch before exercising, and this is very sound advice. The question is, what's the best way to stretch? We believe that the best warm-up method to use before exercising—and closely guarded Eastern bloc sports medicine research from East Germany and the former Soviet Union supports this idea—incorporates joint mobility and dynamic stretching. Joint-mobility exercises and dynamic stretching use the three "Ms"—Movement, Momentum, and Muscular effort—to warm up your joints and muscles to help prevent or decrease the risk of joint trauma and muscle tears and strain. Unlike static stretching, which is slow and constant and in which (traditionally) a muscle is held in a static (nonmoving) position for twenty seconds or longer, joint-mobility and dynamic-stretching exercises involve continuous movements.

The importance of joint-mobility exercises and dynamic stretching is often overlooked, but these activities are crucial for maintaining the integrity of your joints, ligaments, and tendons and your muscle elasticity as you age. These simple exercises help lubricate the joints, improve range of motion, and keep the body functioning optimally by stimulating the circulation of synovial fluid around the joints. We strongly encourage you to include a few of these joint-mobility exercises as part of your warm-up routine.

Simple examples of joint-mobility and dynamic-stretching exercises are arm circles and swings (see below). Several other joint-mobility and dynamic-stretching movements that you can include in your warm-up sessions are offered below.

Arm Swings
1. Stand with your feet shoulder width apart.
2. Relax your arms and shoulders, and swing your arms back and forth across the front of your body.
3. Complete twenty to twenty-five full swings.

Trunk Rotations

1. Stand with your feet shoulder width apart. Place your hands on your hips.
2. Flex your knees slightly and turn from side to side, keeping your feet firmly on the floor. Twist as far as is comfortable.
3. Do twenty to twenty-five complete swings.

Back Stretch

1. Lie on your back on a firm, slightly padded surface (exercise mat, folded blanket, thick rug) and bring both knees to your chest. Clasp your hands behind the back of your knees.
2. Roll forward until your feet touch the floor, and then immediately roll back until your head nearly touches the floor.
3. Complete fifteen to twenty full rolls.

Leg Swings

1. Stand with your feet shoulder width apart.
2. While keeping your upper body perpendicular to the floor, swing one leg forward and backward. Swing your leg as far as you can without allowing your upper body to move.
3. If balance is a problem, you can do this stretching exercise while keeping one hand on top of a chair or table as a precaution. Remember to keep your body perpendicular, however; do not lean.
4. Repeat the swing motion fifteen times on each leg.
5. As a variation, you can swing your leg across the front of your body, which stretches a different set of muscles.

More Advanced Joint Mobility and Dynamic Stretching Exercises

No-Jump Jacks

1. Stand with your feet together and your palms pressing into your outer thighs.
2. Swing your arms straight up over your head and clap your palms together.
3. Return your arms and palms to the starting position. Repeat nine more times.

Bent Shoulder Circles

1. Stand with your feet shoulder width apart, and bend forward at the waist about 45 degrees.
2. Move your right arm as if you were drawing big circles on the floor. "Draw" ten circles with your right arm, then switch to your left arm and "draw" ten circles.
3. Repeat the cycle with first one arm, then the other, four more times. Each time, change the size of the circles you draw.

Knee Hugs

1. Stand upright with your feet comfortably apart for balance.
2. Quickly raise one knee and hug it toward your chest.
3. Lower your leg and repeat with the other knee.
4. Repeat the complete sequence five to ten times.

Reach and Squat

1. Stand upright with your feet slightly wider than your shoulders. Make sure your feet are pointing directly forward.
2. Slowly lower your body into a squat position while keep-

ing your head and chest up and your feet flat on the
ground.

3. As you squat, reach straight up over your shoulders with
both arms.
4. Slowly return to a standing position and lower your
arms.
5. Repeat the sequence five to ten times.

Static Stretching

Static-stretching exercises are more appropriate as part of your
cooldown program after you have finished exercising. You
should always remember to breathe naturally while performing static stretches; do not hold your breath. You can also do
a mixture of dynamic and static stretching as part of your
cooldown.

Chest Stretch

1. Stand with your feet slightly wider than shoulder width
apart. Keep your knees slightly bent.
2. Hold your arms out to the side, parallel with the floor,
with palms facing forward.
3. Stretch your arms back as far as you can, and hold that
position for twenty seconds.
4. Return to the starting position, and repeat the stretch
once more.

Upper Back Stretch

1. Stand with your feet slightly wider than shoulder width
apart, knees slightly bent.
2. Interlock your fingers, turn your palms outward, and
push your hands as far away from your chest as you can.
Hold that position for twenty seconds. Repeat two more
times.

Side Bends

1. Stand with your feet slightly wider than shoulder width apart, knees slightly bent. Place your hands on your hips.
2. Bend slowly to one side, hold the position for twenty seconds, then return to the vertical position.
3. Bend slowly to the other side, hold, then return to the starting position. Repeat both bends two more times. Do not lean backward or forward.

Hamstring Stretch

1. Sit on the floor and place both legs straight out in front of you.
2. Bend your left leg and place the sole of the left foot next to the knee of your right leg. Relax your left leg so that it naturally falls toward the floor.
3. Bend forward while keeping your back straight. You should feel the stretch in your hamstring in your right leg. Hold the position for twenty seconds.
4. Repeat the stretch with the other leg, and hold for twenty seconds.

Calf Stretch

1. Stand in front of a wall, extend both arms, and place your hands flat at shoulder height against the wall. Place one leg in front of the other.
2. Slowly move your back leg away from the wall. Keep it straight, and keep your front leg pressed into the floor.
3. Keep your hips facing the wall and the back leg and spine straight.
4. Hold the stretch for twenty seconds.
5. Return the back leg to the starting position and do the stretch using the other leg. Repeat the entire sequence one more time.

Groin Stretch

1. Sit on the floor and bring both feet toward your body. Place the soles of your feet together, and allow your knees to come up and out to the sides.
2. Rest your hands on your lower legs or ankles and gently ease both knees toward the floor.
3. Hold the stretch for twenty seconds, then relax. Repeat two more times. You will feel the stretch along the inside of your thighs and groin.

THE BOTTOM LINE

"Quality over quantity" is a bit of a cliché, but nevertheless this common dictum rings true with exercise, too. Even a relatively small amount of exercise can reap dividends when it comes to preventing and controlling diabetes, notwithstanding the benefits in terms of stress reduction and overall quality of life that can be traced directly to physical activity.

We leave you with poignant information from two recent scientific studies. In one, the scientists compared two groups of type 2 diabetics: those who exercised for four months and then stopped (controls) and those who continued on for an additional four months. The Hb A_{1c} levels declined in the active patients and increased in the controls. The active patients also benefited from significant declines in triglyceride and total cholesterol levels, while controls had increases in both factors. And in a recent ten-year study, investigators found that diabetics age fifty and older who walked one or more miles per day were half as likely to die of cardiovascular disease or any other causes than diabetics who did not walk.

So stick with it. Keep moving. Live longer and prosper.

Chapter 8

The Power of Natural Supplements

Some of the most exciting—and underutilized—advancements being made in the optimization of healthy blood glucose metabolism involve the use of natural supplements. Ongoing research by innovative scientists is regularly uncovering new options for the prevention and treatment of metabolic diseases, especially regarding the use of certain nutraceuticals. New studies continue to support the favorable impact of supplementation with specific nutraceuticals on gene expression and the enhancement of healthy blood sugar metabolism at a molecular level. Many of the studies focus on the use of nutraceuticals to support beta-cell function, insulin sensitivity, and healthy blood glucose levels. Some of these supplements have a special synergy with prescription medications as well as the antiglycation eating plan that we discussed in chapters 5 and 6. Thus we believe it is vitally important to incorporate nutraceuticals

A food containing health-giving additives and having medicinal benefits

148

into our strategy to support metabolic function, based on your individual needs.

In this chapter, we discuss the role of the most effective scientifically investigated supplements and help you identify which supplements may most benefit you. We have divided the supplements into four basic categories (beta-cell health; insulin sensitizers; antiglycation agents; and antioxidants and anti-inflammatory agents) that mirror the key factors involved in metabolic dysfunction. Understand that the divisions are somewhat artificial, given that nutraceuticals have a fair degree of crossover and complementary effects and health benefits.

As always, talk to your doctor before you begin any nutraceutical program, especially if you are taking any type of medication.

BETA-CELL HEALTH

Beta cells reside in the pancreas, where their primary function is to secrete insulin in response to glucose in the bloodstream. In type 2 diabetes, beta cells are dysfunctional. The following supplements have shown promise for supporting beta-cell health.

Coffee Berries

Your morning cup of coffee started out as a bright red fruit (berry). The coffee berry is rich in antioxidants and other phytonutrients known as polyphenols. These polyphenols (or phenolic acids) have been shown to be helpful in supporting optimal blood glucose levels as well as in fighting damaging free radicals and protecting cardiovascular health. But before you plug in your twelve-cup coffeemaker and get out your 20-ounce coffee mug, you need to look at the *best* way for you to get the benefits from coffee berries.

Several studies suggest that coffee consumption (the coffee beverage is made from the roasted seeds of the coffee berry) helps with blood glucose control and other diabetes-related problems. Results of a twelve-year study of more than twelve thousand middle-aged adults who did not have diabetes at the start of the study found that those who drank four or more cups of coffee daily were one-third less likely to develop type 2 diabetes during the study period. This study, published in December 2006, followed others that reported similar findings, and the studies continue. One study conducted at the University of Minnesota indicated that decaffeinated coffee was better at reducing the risk of diabetes than regular coffee.

Greater power appears to reside in the whole berry, not just in the coffee seed, or bean, which is what remains after the outer layers of the berries are separated out and the beans are roasted. Coffee berries contain polyphenols that have been shown to support healthy blood glucose, cholesterol, and triglyceride levels, and to reduce free-radical damage, among other benefits that are especially important for people with insulin resistance and/or diabetes. Many of these benefits are significantly reduced once the berries are harvested, processed, and roasted to make the cup of coffee you enjoy. Yes, please be aware that glycotoxins are formed during the roasting of coffee beans, and our goal is to limit the ingestion of dietary glycotoxins. Therefore, to reap the optimal positive impact of the entire coffee berry, it's an intelligent strategy to take a supplement that contains all the polyphenols found in the fruit, without all the caffeine and glycotoxins that form from dry roasting coffee beans at high temperatures.

Coffee berries contain some well-studied phytochemicals, such as chlorogenic acid and caffeic acid. Since glucose generation from glycogen stored in the liver is often overactive in people who have high blood sugar, reducing the gene expression of key enzymes involved in this action can lead to reduced blood sugar levels.

That's where chlorogenic acid comes in: it can inhibit the gene expression of an important enzyme involved in generating glucose from glycogen, and thus can reduce glucose production. In a trial at the Moscow Modern Medical Center, seventy-five healthy volunteers were given either 90 mg of chlorogenic acid daily or a placebo. Blood glucose levels of the chlorogenic acid group were 15 to 20 percent lower than those of the placebo group. Scientists have also shown that chlorogenic acid can decrease the absorption rate of glucose.

At National Cheng Kung University in Taiwan, scientists determined that caffeic acid increases glucose uptake into cells, thus removing it from the bloodstream. When researchers at nearby Taipei Medical College injected caffeic acid into diabetic animals, their glucose levels declined.

To enjoy the benefits of coffee berries, look for extracts that are standardized to 50 percent total phenolic acids and 15,000 µmol/g of ORAC (oxygen-radical absorbent capacity). The recommended dosage is 100 mg of extract three times daily.

Ginseng

The term "ginseng" refers to several species of the genus *Panax*, of which the most commonly used are American ginseng (*Panax quinquefolius*) and Asian ginseng (*Panax ginseng*). A third type is Siberian ginseng (*Eleutherococcus senticosus*), which is from a different genus and does not contain the components (ginsenosides) present in the *Panax* species that are believed to give it healing qualities.

For more than two thousand years, practitioners of traditional Chinese medicine have used ginseng root to treat various ailments. It has largely been valued as a way to boost the immune system and as an adaptogen, which means it helps increase the body's resistance to stress. Today it is still used for this purpose, but it also is proving helpful in supporting metabolic health and healthy blood sugar levels.

At the University of Toronto, a group of researchers found that Asian ginseng, when compared with a placebo, improved glucose and insulin control in people with type 2 diabetes. The patients in the double-blind study took 6 g of ginseng (2 g per meal) or a placebo daily, along with their usual diet and/or medications. At the end of three months, the ginseng had significantly improved plasma glucose and fasting plasma insulin levels.

American ginseng (*Panax quinquefolius*) was the center of attention in another study, in which researchers found evidence that the herb prevented the destruction of beta cells. Yet it seems that Asian ginseng also may be helpful, as studies with diabetic animals treated with extracts of *Panax ginseng* show improved blood glucose levels and glucose tolerance, and also weight loss.

Although ginseng roots are traditionally the part of the plant used in remedies, a 2002 study at the University of Chicago found that an extract of the ginseng berry could be useful in treating diabetes and obesity. When the researchers administered ginseng to an experimental test group with diabetes, the group's blood glucose levels, sensitivity to insulin, cholesterol levels, and weight improved, and appetite decreased. The study's investigators concluded that the chemical makeup of the berries differs from that of the root, yet the berries were very effective in treating diabetes.

The recommended dose is 200 mg daily of ginseng extract standardized to 4 percent ginsenosides. In sensitive individuals, the most common side effects are excitability and nervousness, which usually decrease after the first few days. Children and pregnant or nursing women should not take ginseng without their doctor's knowledge, because it has estrogen-like effects.

Vitamin D and Calcium

The scientific data on vitamin D's myriad of beneficial health effects are just starting to accumulate. Beyond bone health, recent studies suggest amazing benefits from vitamin D, including the support of vascular health and powerful anticancer properties.

Vitamin D may play several different roles in metabolic health, one of which is the ability to improve beta-cell function and insulin resistance in type 2 diabetes. The vitamin may also be instrumental in reducing the incidence of type 1 diabetes. The benefit was illustrated in a study, published in *Lancet,* in which investigators followed nearly eleven thousand children for more than ten years. They found that the incidence of diabetes was nearly 80 percent lower in children who had taken 2,000 IU of vitamin D daily during their first year of life compared with children who had not.

When vitamin D supplements are paired with calcium, we see impressive metabolic health improvements as well. In a study of about three hundred adults aged sixty-five or older, a third of whom had prediabetes, Anastassios Pittas, M.D., of the Tufts-New England Medical Center in Boston, found that the fasting blood glucose levels of people with prediabetes rose significantly less over three years if they took 700 IU of vitamin D and 500 mg of calcium daily than if they took a placebo.

In a much larger study, Dr. Pittas and colleagues followed the progress of 83,779 women from the Nurses' Health Study who were free of diabetes, cardiovascular disease, and cancer at the start of the study. During the twenty years of follow-up, the researchers assessed the women's vitamin D and calcium intake every two to four years. The investigators determined that a combined daily intake of more than 1,200 mg calcium and more than 800 IU vitamin D was associated with 33 percent less risk of type 2 diabetes than intakes of less than 600 mg calcium and less than 400 IU vitamin D. Dr. Pittas and his team reported in 2007 the results of a meta-analysis in which they noted that supplementing with both vitamin D and calcium can have a beneficial impact on glucose metabolism in people with type 2 diabetes.

Another possible link between vitamin D and diabetes is the fact that being overweight or obese increases the body's need for the vitamin. Since vitamin D is, in fact, a fat-soluble hormone, it is stored in fat tissue, leaving less available in the bloodstream.

INSULIN SENSITIZERS

The more sensitive or receptive your cells are to insulin, the better you can control your blood glucose levels and in turn reduce your risk of developing diabetic complications. The following supplements have been shown to increase insulin sensitivity.

Barley Extract

Barley extract contains beta-glucan, a naturally derived fiber that has a sticky, glutinous consistency. The stickiness of beta-glucan slows down the absorption of glucose into the bloodstream and helps to optimize blood glucose levels. Barley extract also reduced Hb A_{1c} and fasting blood glucose in experimental studies. To reduce total and LDL cholesterol levels and increase HDL cholesterol, human clinical data suggest that a dose of 15 per day is effective in both people with high cholesterol and those who have type 2 diabetes.

Swiss researchers report that a 50 percent reduction in peak glycemic values can be achieved when diabetics eat a concentration of 10 percent beta-glucan in a cereal food, and that LDL cholesterol can also be significantly reduced with a daily intake of 3 g or more of beta-glucan.

In one study, seventy-five men and women with high cholesterol took either 6 g of concentrated beta-glucan or a placebo daily for six weeks. The patients who took the beta-glucan experienced a significant reduction in total and LDL cholesterol over the control patients, suggesting this dose may be helpful in people who are at risk for cardiovascular disease.

Claudia, a fifty-two-year-old graphic artist, was no stranger to barley, as she had been including it in her diet occasionally as part of her efforts to control her glucose levels with an antiglycation diet and exercise. When her fasting glucose levels began to creep up to 125 mg/dL and higher, she asked about taking barley extract instead of considering medication. She started with 6 g of barley extract daily, and after one month, her fasting glucose levels were consistently less than 115 mg/dL, and a lipid panel revealed a ten-point drop in her total cholesterol. "I'm really pleased with the results," she said. "I'm adding more barley extract and soluble oat fiber to my diet as well, and I'm hoping I can really bring my glucose levels down to optimal levels." Six months later, her fasting glucose levels were often close to 100 mg/dL, and her total cholesterol also dropped below 200.

A small percentage of people are hypersensitive to barley, especially those with celiac disease. If you have celiac disease or are sensitive to wheat, rye, or other grains that contain gluten, use barley and barley extract cautiously.

Carnitine

Carnitine is a derivative of the amino acids lysine and methionine. It is involved in energy production and specifically assists with the oxidation of glucose. Several published scientific studies have shown that carnitine supplementation supports insulin sensitivity and optimizes blood glucose levels. Carnitine has also been shown to decrease fat levels in muscle.

A study conducted by experts at Wayne State University in Detroit, Michigan, showed the benefits of taking carnitine for metabolic health. The researchers examined data from two yearlong, placebo-controlled trials that involved more than 1,200 patients with diabetes. They found that patients who took 500 to 1,000 mg of carnitine three times a day had significant improvements in pain and also experienced improved nerve-fiber regeneration and vibration perception, all of which are related to diabetic neuropathy.

An experimental study recently showed that carnitine also has antiglycation powers. Scientists fed large amounts of fructose to the animals in the experiment and treated some of the group with carnitine. The supplement significantly reduced glycation and the accumulation of AGEs in the treated experimental group.

When it comes to the cardiovascular system and the heart, carnitine supplementation is very helpful. A recent study, published in *Drugs and Experimental Clinical Research,* showed that carnitine supplementation improved quality of life and life expectancy in patients who had suffered a heart attack. Another study, published in *American Heart Journal,* indicated improvements in survival associated with carnitine supplementation in patients with heart failure. These studies and many others support carnitine's role in protecting and enhancing cardiovascular health. A number of other experimental studies in aging animals and other test models suggest carnitine may be beneficial in preventing age-related declines in memory and energy metabolism. For example, a recent study, published in *Proceedings of the National Academy of Sciences,* showed that supplementing with lipoic acid and acetyl-L-carnitine (a form of carnitine particularly good for brain health) reversed energy deficits in the brains of experimental animals. A 2006 study, published in *Biogerontology,* showed that carnitine and lipoic acid dramatically improved heart muscle energy production. Yet another recent experimental study, published in *Mechanisms of Ageing and Development,* showed that carnitine decreased age-induced dysfunction in aging heart muscle.

The suggested dose of carnitine (as L-carnitine, acetyl-L-carnitine, or propionyl-L-carnitine) is 2,000 mg daily. Side effects are uncommon but may include diarrhea or stomach pain.

Chromium

Chromium is a nutrient that is essential for fat and carbohydrate metabolism. It also aids in insulin metabolism, and thus may reduce insulin resistance. It also serves as a coenzyme for several different enzymes.

The U.S. Department of Agriculture reports that most Americans fail to consume enough chromium in their diets. In fact, most diets contain less than 60 percent of the minimum suggested amount (50 micrograms [μg or mcg]) of chromium daily. This fact is especially important if you are concerned about prediabetes or already have diabetes, because insufficient levels of chromium can lead to signs and symptoms similar to those associated with diabetes and cardiovascular disease, including an increase in blood sugar, triglyceride, and cholesterol levels. Fortunately, many studies show that chromium supplements taken by people who have low chromium levels and who also are diabetic or have impaired glucose tolerance can result in improvements in blood glucose, insulin, and lipid levels.

In 2006, scientists published a comprehensive review of many studies involving nearly 1,700 patients who took chromium and concluded that the mineral was very helpful in supporting healthy blood glucose, insulin, cholesterol, and triglyceride levels as well as in reducing the need for oral diabetes medications.

Proper dosing of chromium is important if you want to get the most benefit. In 1997, a study published in *Diabetes* compared the effects of two different doses—1,000 mcg and 200 mcg—and a placebo. Among patients who took 1,000 mcg, Hb A$_{1c}$ values improved significantly after two months, and it improved in both treatment groups after four months. Patients who took the higher dose of chromium also experienced lower fasting glucose levels.

Not all studies of the effects of chromium on insulin resistance, blood glucose levels, and diabetes in general have yielded positive results, largely due to the inadequate dosages used in the trials. It is hoped that additional studies will help resolve questions about chromium use in diabetes. One study that could help in this regard is currently ongoing and headed by the diabetes expert William T. Cefalu, M.D. This National Institutes of Health four-year study is evaluating the use of 1,000 mcg of chromium per day in people who have type 2 diabetes.

The dosing of chromium recommended by the Institute of Medicine is 35 mcg for men and 25 mcg for women ages nineteen to fifty years; 30 mcg for men and 20 mcg for women fifty-one years and older; and 30 mcg for pregnant or breast-feeding women nineteen years and older. We have had excellent results with a suggested dosage of 600 to 1,000 mcg daily.

Cinnamon

Since the dawn of human civilization, the aromatic spice cinnamon has been used to enhance food flavor and to manage various health conditions. Recently, however, cinnamon has been recognized for its remarkable effects on glucose metabolism.

Researchers at the U.S. Department of Agriculture's Beltsville Human Nutrition Research Center found that cinnamon contains certain water-soluble compounds—known collectively as polyphenols—that can increase glucose metabolism, which helps lower blood sugar levels and fight free-radical damage. Cinnamon can also help reduce lipid levels while improving glucose metabolism, which is an ideal combination for fighting metabolic problems and cardiovascular disease. For example, in a recent clinical study, adults with type 2 diabetes were given either a placebo or 1 g, 3 g, or 6 g of cinnamon daily for forty days. At the end of the forty-day period, the patients who had taken cinnamon had significantly reduced levels of fasting serum glucose, total cholesterol, low-density lipoprotein (LDL), and triglycerides, and the reduction was greater as the dose of cinnamon increased. For twenty days after the end of treatment, the triglyceride and glucose levels continued to stay low, while LDL and total cholesterol levels continued to decline.

"I admit I was skeptical, but I figured I had nothing to lose by trying the cinnamon supplements," says Bonnie, a forty-eight-year-old antiques dealer. She had been only partly successful in controlling her blood glucose levels with diet and exercise, and her total cholesterol level had stubbornly remained around 230 mg/dL, despite her careful dietary efforts. In April she began taking 2 g of cinnamon extract every day, and by the end of May, her cholesterol had dropped to 212 mg/dL, and her fasting glucose had declined from around 145 mg/dL to an average of 130 mg/dL.

The number of studies documenting the effectiveness of cinnamon in diabetes continues to grow. The polyphenols in cinnamon were recently found to not only increase insulin-dependent glucose metabolism by roughly twentyfold but also to act as antioxidants. Moreover, scientists at Iowa State University determined that these polyphenols have a positive impact on gene expression, which ultimately results in a decline in blood glucose levels.

The recommended dose of cinnamon is 125 mg of water-soluble cinnamon extract standardized to 0.95 percent trimeric and tetrameric A-type polymers (1.2 mg) taken three times daily. A water-soluble cinnamon extract is preferred over taking 3 to 6 g of whole cinnamon because of concerns regarding the chronic ingestion of volatile compounds, such as aldehydes, alcohols, and esters, which are found in whole cinnamon and have the potential to cause chromosome damage.

Curcumin

The exotic aromas and flavors of Indian and some Asian cuisines owe much to turmeric, a spice that also has potent antioxidant and anti-inflammatory properties. Curcumin, a component of the turmeric root, is the key mediator of these beneficial properties. Curcumin has been shown in a great number of studies to possess remarkable qualities, including an ability to inhibit the development of diabetic retinopathy and diabetic nephropathy in experimental models, as well as to protect the nervous and cardiovascular systems and support a healthy colon.

The results of studies involving curcumin and diabetes have been very encouraging. In one experimental model, a diabetic test group was given curcumin for forty-five days and had a significant decrease in blood glucose levels. In another study, curcumin inhibited the development of diabetic retinopathy. Curcumin has also suppressed the formation of cataracts in experimental models by providing protection against the ravages of runaway glycation. There is also good experimental evidence that curcumin supports the function of insulin-producing pancreatic beta cells.

To take advantage of curcumin's multiple health benefits,

we recommend you take at least 800 mg daily of turmeric (*Curcuma longa*) root extract standardized for 95 percent curcuminoids. Recently, higher bioavailable formulations of curcumin have been studied and should be available in the near future.

Before trying curcumin, tell your doctor if you are taking any blood-thinning medications (such as warfarin, aspirin), if you are pregnant or breast-feeding, or if you have gallstones, an ulcer, or liver or bile obstruction. Side effects are rare.

DHEA

Dehydroepiandrosterone (DHEA), which is manufactured in the body and secreted by the adrenal glands, has been called the "mother of all hormones" because it serves as a precursor to both male and female sex hormones, such as testosterone and estrogen. Actually, that label is somewhat inaccurate, because cholesterol serves as the key starting point for the production of all sex hormones. Today, DHEA is perhaps best known for its role in aging.

DHEA levels in the body begin to decline after age thirty. Along with aging, declining levels of DHEA are associated with higher glucose levels. Research suggests that DHEA improves glucose metabolism by increasing glucose uptake by cells as well as by decreasing the gene expression of certain enzymes involved in glucose production in the liver. Experimental studies in both animals and humans show that DHEA supplementation improves insulin sensitivity and reduces obesity, while other animal studies indicate that DHEA increases beta-cell mass and improves glucose-dependent insulin secretion in aging.

Published study data indicate that testosterone improves insulin sensitivity in men. This suggests that DHEA's conversion into testosterone may be at least partly responsible for the beneficial effects it has on insulin function.

Before you take DHEA, consult with your health-care provider so he or she can determine the optimal dose for you. We strongly recommend that you have your DHEA levels checked several weeks after starting supplementation to make sure your levels are in an optimal range. The typical dose for DHEA supplementation is 15 to 75 mg daily, taken in the early morning.

Magnesium

People with metabolic dysfunction and diabetes are very often deficient in magnesium. Magnesium is used by all the cells in the body and is especially involved in supporting the relationship between glucose metabolism and insulin. Low levels or an obvious deficiency can worsen insulin resistance. Research clearly supports the benefits of magnesium supplementation on glucose metabolism. For example, a 2003 study published in the journal *Diabetes Care* shows that magnesium supplementation in patients with type 2 diabetes significantly improved insulin sensitivity, blood glucose control, and blood pressure.

Strong evidence in support of magnesium supplementation and its role in metabolic health is found in several large studies that evaluated data from more than 170,000 people. Several studies conducted at Harvard University show that high dietary magnesium intake is associated with a significantly reduced risk of developing type 2 diabetes, even in people who are obese. In one of these studies, the length of follow-up was twelve to eighteen years.

In another study that followed more than 4,600 people aged eighteen to thirty, the researchers found that those who consumed the most magnesium had the least risk of developing metabolic syndrome. A greater intake of magnesium was associated with a reduced risk of having high blood glucose levels, low levels of "good" cholesterol, or excess fat around the waist. And in yet another large study (more than 25,000 participants followed for ten years), a combination of soluble fiber and magnesium appeared to be effective in decreasing the risk of type 2 diabetes. Magnesium also appears to be an important factor in reducing the risk of diabetic retinopathy, as a deficiency of this mineral was found to be significantly associated with this dreaded complication.

The recommended dose of magnesium to support metabolic health is 160 mg three times daily, preferably as magnesium citrate. Consult your doctor before taking magnesium supplements if you have myasthenia gravis or kidney failure.

Omega-3 Fatty Acids

Omega-3 fatty acids are essential fatty acids, which means your body needs them but cannot manufacture them. This means you must get these nutrients from your diet and/or through dietary supplementation. Omega-3 fatty acids are found in relatively high levels in certain fish and seafood, as well as in some plant sources (see chapter 5).

An apparent paradox is the fact that although the native Inuit people get an enormous amount of fat in their diet from fish, whales, and seals, they do not suffer a correspondingly high rate of heart attacks. At least part of the reason for this phenomenon is that they consume high levels of omega-3 fatty acids, which reduce the blood's tendency to coagulate and form clots while simultaneously optimizing blood cholesterol and lipid levels, all important benefits in the context of diabetes.

The three major types of omega-3s found in foods and used by the body are alpha-linolenic acid (ALA), eicosapentaenoic acid (EPA), and docosahexaenoic acid (DHA). When you eat foods that contain ALA, your body converts it to EPA and

DHA. Unfortunately, the conversion process becomes inefficient as we age, so it is ideal to obtain DHA and EPA directly when possible.

An enormous body of research shows that omega-3s help reduce inflammation, support ideal triglyceride and HDL cholesterol levels, and reduce blood pressure, all of which are very important for maintaining cardiovascular and metabolic health. These fatty acids also enhance glucose metabolism, reduce C-reactive protein levels, and support fat metabolism, factors closely linked to complications associated with diabetes.

In a National Eye Institute and National Institutes of Health study, for example, investigators found that omega-3 fatty acids promoted the health of and protected against diseases of the retina, which supports their use in helping to prevent diabetic retinopathy. Recent studies also suggest that omega-3s slow the progression of plaque accumulation in women who have diabetes and coronary artery disease. The ability of omega-3 fatty acids to significantly reduce the risk of sudden cardiac death—by 45 percent—was demonstrated in the GISSI Prevention study, in which more than eleven thousand patients participated.

A recent review of the use of omega-3 fatty acids in the treatment of hypertension found that omega-3s protect against stroke and reaffirmed that the cardioprotective benefits of omega-3 fatty acids are related to their ability to improve blood pressure, vascular function, lipid metabolism, inflammation, and cardiac function. It appears that DHA is more beneficial when it comes to reducing blood pressure and heart rate, as well as improving vascular function.

We strongly recommend that for optimal metabolic and cardiovascular health, you consume at least 1,400 mg of EPA and 1,000 mg of DHA daily. The most convenient way to accomplish this is to consume a high-quality fish oil certified by

International Fish Oil Standards (www.nutrasource.ca/ifos_new/ index.asp) to be free of toxins such as heavy metals (mercury, cadmium), PCBs, dioxins, and fluoranes. You can and should consume more ALA from sources such as walnuts and flaxseed, but know that its rate of conversion to EPA and DHA becomes inefficient as we age.

ANTIGLYCATION AGENTS

Preventing glycation is one of the main goals of everyone concerned with reducing the risk of diabetes-related complications as well as premature aging. Along with intelligent food preparation/cooking methods that reduce dietary glycotoxin ingestion, there are several dietary supplements that can be a helpful part of an antiglycation strategy.

Benfotiamine

Glycotoxins damage your body at both the macrovascular and microvascular level. To help protect yourself against the damaging consequences of glycation, there's one supplement that is especially important: benfotiamine.

Few people have heard about this special variation of vitamin B_1, which has been shown to prevent nerve *and* blood vessel damage—and the resulting complications—that are caused by glycation. Many experimental studies show that benfotiamine relieves pain due to the nerve and inflammatory damage wrought by glycation, helps alleviate oxidative damage, and prevents glycation-induced damage to the all-important endothelium in blood vessels. For example, a recent study showed that the supplement significantly improved blood flow and reduced oxidative stress in patients with type 2 diabetes who were given meals high in food-derived glycotoxins.

A study recently published in *Diabetes Care* showed the amazing effect of benfotiamine on preventing glycotoxin-induced inflammation, endothelial dysfunction in the vascular system, and oxidative stress in human patients with type 2 diabetes. In this important study, patients with type 2 diabetes were given a heat-processed test meal with a high level of dietary glycotoxins and then supplemented with 1,050 mg of benfotiamine daily. Benfotiamine significantly reduced glycotoxin-induced damage to the vascular system in these patients.

Another impressive study in patients with diabetes-induced painful peripheral neuropathy showed that 100 mg of benfotiamine given four times daily significantly improved neuropathy scores, with the greatest effect being a reduction in pain in these patients. This recent study confirmed the results of a 1999 study that showed significant improvements in neuropathy scores after only three weeks in type 2 diabetic patients suffering from painful peripheral diabetic neuropathy. These patients received up to 320 mg of benfotiamine daily, with greater benefits seen in the high-dose group.

Benfotiamine provides tremendous benefit by stopping the accumulation of sugar-derived compounds called triosephosphates that gather in blood and nerve cells and damage them. Benfotiamine activates the enzyme transketolase, which in turn makes triosephosphates into harmless chemicals, inhibiting the damaging action of glycation. We strongly believe that benfotiamine supplementation is very beneficial for patients who have diabetic neuropathy, diabetic retinopathy, and kidney disease.

In a recent study, a daily dose of 1,050 mg of benfotiamine dramatically reduced endothelial and oxidative damage in patients who were on high-glycotoxin diets. Lower doses have shown benefit in type 2 diabetic patients in the context of painful peripheral diabetic neuropathy. No side effects have been reported from the use of benfotiamine.

Carnosine and Its Precursors

Carnosine is a molecule (dipeptide) composed of two amino acids, beta-alanine and histidine. Carnosine is valuable because it helps inhibit accelerated aging by interfering with glycation, thus protecting against glycation-induced damage and acting as an antioxidant to fight oxidative stress.

Evidence of carnosine's antiglycation abilities has been seen in several studies. In one recent example involving human cell cultures, carnosine protected against damage to kidney cells from high glucose levels. In another, investigators noted that carnosine and its two precursors—beta-alanine and histidine—may help inhibit the development of atherosclerosis caused by high levels of glycation in diabetes. In addition to its ability to bind to protein molecules and act as a shield against sugar molecules, thus preventing glycation, carnosine can also stimulate enzymes and other substances to eliminate damaged, glycated protein. In these ways, carnosine helps reduce the impact of diabetic complications. When carnosine has been compared with the antiglycating drug aminoguanidine, the supplement has proved to be similarly effective, likely because it inhibits glycation earlier in the process than does the drug.

Some researchers have discounted carnosine's antiglycation abilities because enzymes in the gastrointestinal (GI) tract can degrade this molecule. However, a review of the scientific literature clearly shows that carnosine can be absorbed intact through the GI tract. Furthermore, carnosine's precursors, beta-alanine and histidine, have been shown in a number of studies to boost carnosine levels, so if there are any lingering concerns about direct carnosine supplementation, beta-alanine and histidine can be used instead.

The suggested dosage of carnosine for patients with diabetes is at least 1,000 mg daily and preferably 3,000 to 6,000 mg daily, or comparable amounts of beta-alanine and histidine. No side effects have been noted.

ANTIOXIDANTS AND ANTI-INFLAMMATORY AGENTS

Antioxidants provide a critical defense against the damage caused by excess oxidative stress. Free radical–inspired oxidative damage accelerates aging and contributes to many diseases, including diabetes, cancer, arthritis, and heart disease. Anti-inflammatory strategies are important for fighting the damage caused by glycation and the production of inflammatory substances (cytokines) that can lead to endothelial vascular damage. Glycotoxins derived from foods cooked with intense heat under dry conditions contribute to both oxidative damage as well as inflammation. For example, a 2002 study, published in *Proceedings of the National Academy of Sciences,* showed that over six weeks, a diet high in glycotoxins increased the level of C-reactive protein (CRP) by 20 percent and the proinflammatory cytokine tumor necrosis factor-alpha by 86 percent in diabetic patients. Research also shows that diabetes prompts white blood cells to release proinflammatory chemicals that can significantly damage the delicate vascular endothelial cells. A study published by researchers at the Mount Sinai School of Medicine in April 2007 showed that dietary glycotoxins correlated with oxidative stress, inflammation of blood vessels, and insulin resistance. For these and many other reasons, it is important that you follow an antiglycation diet and complement that effort with natural supplements.

Alpha-Lipoic Acid

Alpha-lipoic acid (ALA) has been approved for the prevention and treatment of diabetic neuropathy in Germany for nearly thirty years. In addition, this potent antioxidant has been shown to offer impressive protection against glycation- and aging-induced damage to the heart and blood vessels, kidneys, and nerves. In one study, for example, patients who suffered painful diabetic neuropathy experienced significant improvement after taking 600 mg of ALA daily for five weeks. In another study, patients with type 2 diabetes took 600 mg of alpha-lipoic acid daily for three months. At the end of the study, twenty patients had a significant improvement in their neuropathic symptoms, and five patients had no more symptoms at all.

Olivia, a sixty-one-year-old retired high school teacher, had been experiencing some painful neuropathy in her right leg. At age fifty-five, she was diagnosed with type 2 diabetes, and for the past three years she had been taking an oral antidiabetes drug. The pain in her leg started gradually, and at first she chose to ignore it and did not mention it to her doctor. Once it affected her daily walks, however, she became concerned, because she was unable to exercise. She insisted that she did not want to take another drug in addition to the metformin she was already taking, so she began taking 600 mg of alpha-lipoic acid daily. After six weeks, she noted an improvement, and two months later, the pain was minimal. She was able to return to her daily walks and eventually lost the few extra pounds she had gained during the time she had stopped walking.

Alpha-lipoic acid's ability to improve blood flow is another impressive attribute that helps in the battle against neuropathy and other diabetic complications. Alpha-lipoic acid also may protect beta cells from oxidative damage.

Alpha-lipoic acid comes in two different chemical forms (isomers)—R and S. Alpha-lipoic acid supplements consist of the R and S form in equal amounts. The human body normally produces and uses R-lipoic acid. This form significantly reduces inflammatory reactions, is more potent than the combined R and S forms, and can revert various antioxidants back to their active states.

Yet another form of lipoic acid that occurs in the body is a variation of the R form: R-dihydro-lipoic acid (R-DHLA). Some health benefits appear to be specific to R-DHLA.

The suggested dose of alpha-lipoic acid is 600 mg daily; for the preferred R-DHLA supplement, it is 150 mg to 300 mg daily. When using lipoic acid for diabetic neuropathy, improvement is usually apparent within three to six weeks.

Coenzyme Q10

Coenzyme Q10 (CoQ10) is a fat-soluble, vitamin-like nutrient that is produced by the body and is present in every cell. This nutrient plays a critical role in energy production and also acts as a potent antioxidant. Levels of CoQ10 decline with age and are also low in people who have diabetes and other chronic conditions, including heart disease and cancer. Food sources include organ meats (such as liver, kidney), beef, soybean oil, mackerel, and peanuts, but the amounts of CoQ10 in food are quite low. Recent scientific research strongly supports the health benefits of ingesting relatively high levels of CoQ10, and for this reason, supplementation is recommended.

CoQ10 exists in two chemically different forms, ubiquinol and ubiquinone. The vast majority of CoQ10 supplements available today contain the ubiquinone form. However, ubiquinol has the ability to scavenge free radicals in sites where inflammation and oxidation caused by glycation can inflict significant damage. Ubiquinol also is the dominant form in most human tissues, as noted in a study published in 1994 in the scientific journal *Molecular Aspects of Medicine.*

Extensive experimental research has shown ubiquinol to be superior and more available to the body than the ubiquinone form found in most commercially available CoQ10 supplements. Recent research published by the CoQ10 expert Peter Langsjoen, M.D., suggests that CoQ10 blood levels for individuals with cardiovascular health concerns (including people with type 2 diabetes) need to be greater than 3.5 mcg/mL for optimal benefit. A recent clinical trial published in the scientific journal *Regulatory and Toxicology Pharmacology* showed that supplementing with just 150 mg per day of ubiquinol resulted in CoQ10 blood levels of 3.84 mcg/mL, while subjects who took 300 mg daily reached levels of 7.28 mcg/mL. It took only four weeks to achieve these desirable high levels.

These data can be contrasted with recently published data in the scientific journals *Archives of Neurology* and *Experimental Neurology,* which showed that much higher doses of ubiquinone were required to obtain comparable blood CoQ10 levels. Specifically, the studies with ubiquinone used 1,200 mg per day to achieve blood concentrations of 3.96 mcg/mL and 2,400 mg per day to reach blood levels of 7.25 mcg/mL.

Scientists have long known that CoQ10 levels decrease with age and that there is a clear association between that decline and age-related problems related to energy production in cells. We also know that ubiquinol has impressive effects on aging. Some of those effects were demonstrated in a 2006 study of experimental aging in animals, published in *Experimental Gerontology.*

Scientists use animals for these types of aging experiments because such studies in humans would take three decades or longer to show results. In this study, two-month-old mice were divided into three groups and fed either standard food (control group), chow fortified with ubiquinone, or chow fortified with ubiquinol. At age three months, the aging rate increased sharply in the control group, while mice receiving ubiquinol or ubiquinone aged at a slower rate. At mouse middle age (nine months), the treated mice were aging at about a 45-percent slower rate than the controls.

Most interesting is what occurred beginning at ten months. That's when the ubiquinol-fed mice were aging 51 percent slower than the placebo group and 40 percent slower than the ubiquinone group. At twelve months of age, mice receiving ubiquinol were healthy and energetic, whereas mice receiving ubiquinone or the placebo had similar signs of degenerative changes and aging. The mice who had received ubiquinol showed a 22-percent slower rate of aging.

Recommended doses of ubiquinol are 50 to 300 mg daily. Achieving comparable blood levels with ubiquinone, even formulations that use enhanced absorption technologies, requires far greater dosages.

French Melon Extract

Superoxide dismutase (SOD) is a naturally occurring enzyme that is a potent antioxidant, helping to protect against free radicals bent on wreaking havoc on your cells. It is especially active against the superoxide radical, one of the most destructive reactive molecules in nature and a significant cause of oxidative stress and inflammation. As SOD levels decline with age, your body increasingly loses the ability to fight the onslaught of free radical–initiated damage. Since diabetes is associated with excess inflammation, oxidation, and glycation, maintaining optimal SOD levels is very important, especially because diabetes is associated with a very high risk of heart attack and stroke due to endothelial dysfunction and atherosclerosis.

Until very recently, oral supplements of SOD have been poorly bioavailable because the molecular structure of the enzyme is easily degraded in the stomach. Now, a specially formulated extract called GliSODin that uses a special protein called gliadin from a fruit source of SOD (a melon called *Cucumis melo*), has become available. This new formulation is absorbed intact, without being destroyed. Remarkable new research from the French National Association for Medical Prevention showed that oral supplementation with GliSODin caused the regression of atherosclerosis in high-risk middle-aged adults. It bears repeating that in this study, atherosclerosis progression was actually *reversed*—not slowed or halted.

Basically, the three-year study included adults (aged forty to forty-six) who had risk factors for metabolic syndrome. Patients who took 500 mg of GliSODin daily and also followed a healthy, Mediterranean-type diet had a significant improvement in their antioxidant levels and, more important, a reversal of intima-media thickness (IMT), a marker of atherosclerosis. Controls who were not taking GliSODin but who were following the diet showed indications of atherosclerosis progression.

The suggested dose of GliSODin is 500 mg daily. Because GliSODin contains wheat protein, do not use this supplement if you are allergic to wheat gluten.

Green Tea

Green tea contains potent antioxidant and polyphenol compounds called catechins, which have been shown to enhance energy in human clinical trials, help balance glucose levels, and protect against the development of atherosclerosis. Study results suggest that the polyphenols in green tea may interfere with the absorption of cholesterol in the intestinal tract and promote its elimination from the body. One catechin in particular, epigallocatechin gallate (EGCG), has been shown in experimental models to possibly enhance insulin action, reduce the formation and growth of fat cells, promote glucose metabolism, and reduce cholesterol and triglyceride levels. Especially promising are the results of several studies in which EGCG helped prevent the destruction of beta cells and others done in diabetic animals in which green tea extract inhibited glycation and the formation of glycotoxins.

The recommended dose of green tea extract is 725 mg daily. When looking for a green tea extract, choose one that provides a minimum of 93 percent polyphenols. A typical cup of green tea contains 50 to 150 mg of polyphenols. Some types of green tea extract contain caffeine. If you are sensitive to the small amount of caffeine in green tea supplements, a decaffeinated extract may be more suitable.

Pomegranate

This unusual, thick-skinned fruit with its hundreds of red seeds provides a juice that contains levels of phytochemicals/antioxidants that are much higher than in the juice of other fruits. The phytochemicals in pomegranates, called punicalagins, have been shown in a number of experimental studies to support optimal blood pressure levels, enhance antioxidant levels, and decrease the risk of vascular endothelial damage associated with diabetes.

Israeli researchers, for example, found that patients with type 2 diabetes who drank pomegranate juice for three months dramatically reduced their intima-media thickness (IMT), an indicator of atherosclerosis. In a study published in 2006 in *Atherosclerosis,* pomegranate juice demonstrated potent antioxidant effects. In another study of patients with type 2 diabetes, concentrated pomegranate juice significantly reduced total cholesterol, low-density lipoprotein cholesterol (LDL), and the ratio of total to high-density lipoprotein cholesterol, all positive developments in helping reduce the risks of complications related to diabetes.

To avoid the fructose and calories found in pomegranate juice, pomegranate extracts are available. If you choose to use pomegranate extract rather than pomegranate juice, look for supplements that are standardized for punicalagins and provide about 78 mg per day—this is the approximate level of polyphenols that showed remarkable, atherosclerosis-reducing properties in the clinical studies.

Whey Protein Isolate

Whey is a protein found in milk. Studies indicate that whey protein can be useful in several ways when it comes to diabetes. Researchers concluded that the people with type 2 diabetes who added whey protein to their high-carbohydrate meals experienced less pronounced blood glucose increases after eating. In another study, whey protein was added to meals that contained rapidly digested and absorbed carbohydrates. The whey protein helped balance insulin secretion with blood glucose levels.

Whey protein also appears to support optimal blood pressure levels and to boost the function of the immune system by enhancing glutathione levels, a powerful endogenous antioxidant remarkable for its liver-detoxifying properties. In fact, glutathione is *the* main antioxidant in the liver, which is the primary organ responsible for processing toxins in the body. Low levels of glutathione are seen in people suffering from oxidative stress, liver disease, and diabetes. Therefore it is important to maintain healthy levels of glutathione in your fight against diabetes and against aging.

Whey protein also appears to be beneficial for weight loss. A hormone called cholecystokinin (CCK) is one cause of the feeling of satisfaction/fullness/satiety you experience after eating. Two university-based studies found that whey protein has a beneficial influence on cholecystokinin. In both studies, participants who consumed whey protein said they experienced a greater sense of satisfaction and fullness than subjects who ate casein, another type of dairy protein. The investigators concluded that whey protein appears to be a valuable supplement for people who need to lose weight.

In yet another experimental study, a test group fed whey protein experienced increased insulin sensitivity and a 40-percent reduction in plasma insulin concentration when compared with beef-fed rats. Both of these findings are associated with improved blood glucose levels and reduced fat storage. The studies' researchers concluded that whey appears to be an excellent protein source that supports healthy blood glucose levels and promotes weight loss.

We recommend a quality, low temperature–processed whey protein isolate that retains all the key functional biological proteins of whey, including immune-boosting lactoferrin (a protein found in milk that acts as an antioxidant and fights inflammation). Dosing is usually 20 to 40 g of whey protein isolate daily, with greater amounts suggested if you are under physical stress (e.g., intense physical exercise), have a serious medical illness or infection, or if your body weight exceeds 200 pounds.

THE BOTTOM LINE

Natural supplements are essential components of a comprehensive metabolic health strategy, along with diet, exercise, and other lifestyle efforts. Our experience has taught us that many patients are able to significantly reduce their dependence on diabetes medication after they incorporate our multifaceted approach to optimize their metabolic health. We strongly urge you to speak with a health-care professional in depth when contemplating integrating nutraceuticals with other diabetes interventions.

Chapter 9

Lifestyle: Living With and Without Diabetes

The jury is in: stress, depression, and other psychological conditions have a direct and significant impact on blood sugar control and metabolic health. Research shows that stress hormones can negatively impact blood glucose and insulin levels.

All of this is actually good news, because you have the power to do something about it. Stress doesn't have to take over your life or ruin your metabolic health. In fact, *right now* you possess everything you need to eliminate the stress and other negative psychological factors that can play havoc with your glucose, insulin, blood pressure, cholesterol, and hormone levels.

With that in mind, we want to help you identify and eliminate the depression, anxiety, and/or stress that is having a negative impact on your health. We will explain ways for you to manage these negative factors in positive ways and will encourage you to make one or more of the techniques we describe a regular part of your life.

DIABETES AND DEPRESSION

Shortly after Jessica was diagnosed with type 2 diabetes, she became depressed. "My grandmother had diabetes, and so does my mother," says the forty-five-year-old real estate broker. "My mother has cataracts, and now she has to use a walker because of the nerve damage and pain in her legs. I look at her and think, 'that's going to be me in a few years.' I feel like I'm doomed."

Jessica isn't alone: people with diabetes are twice as likely to develop depression as people who don't have diabetes. It is estimated that up to 15 percent of people with diabetes have a major depressive disorder and that 25 percent of diabetics experience depressive symptoms at some point. It's also been shown that depression significantly reduces the quality of life of people who have type 2 diabetes.

Many people who are newly diagnosed with diabetes go through a mourning process not unlike that experienced by people who lose a loved one. The stages of mourning include denial, anger, depression, and acceptance.

Jessica, for example, felt a sense of hopelessness because she believed that her family history of diabetes meant she couldn't do anything about changing her future. She also felt angry.

"I was actually angry with myself, because I should have known I was at risk," she says. "I was overweight, I didn't get much exercise, and I had a strong family history of the disease. And I was in a state of denial for a long time, because I avoided getting screened for diabetes. I was afraid of the results."

A Serious Unrecognized Problem

In fact, denial is one reason why depression often goes undiagnosed in diabetics, as many people with diabetes who feel depressed never tell their health-care practitioners. At the same time, however, many physicians never ask about or screen for depression, and so the condition goes underdiagnosed. This is especially unfortunate because the recognition and proper treatment of the problem can not only eliminate depression but also lead to significant improvement in compliance with behavior that can result in better management of the disease.

Depression impacts other diabetes-related issues besides blood sugar control. Accelerated rates of coronary artery disease, for example, have been associated with depression in diabetes. In a four-year study conducted at Duke University, which evaluated more than nine hundred patients with type 2 diabetes and/or depression, researchers found that a combination of diabetes, depression, and heart disease can increase a patient's risk of death by 20 to 30 percent. The results of this 2007 study suggest that diabetes and depression exacerbate each other, but we need more research to identify exactly the reason(s) for this association.

Another problem that affects diabetics who are depressed is that they often fail to take proper care of themselves because of their low mood. It is not unusual for people with prediabetes or type 2 diabetes who are depressed to eat junk food, skip meals, not exercise, and forget to monitor their blood glucose levels. Like Jessica, they feel hopeless, that whatever they do will not make a significant difference. Nothing could be further from the truth.

Treating Depression Without Drugs: Cognitive-Behavioral Therapy

For many years, it was widely believed that antidepressants were the only effective, initial treatment for people who suffered from moderate to severe depression. Recent studies, however, are proving that wrong. Cognitive-behavioral therapy, in fact, can be just as effective as medication.

ARE YOU DEPRESSED?

Very often, people with major depression don't realize they are depressed. If you are experiencing three or more of the following symptoms, or if you have only one or two but you have been feeling that way for two weeks or longer, you should seek help for depression.

- Loss of pleasure or satisfaction in activities you used to enjoy, including sex
- Persistent sadness and/or feelings of pessimism
- Changes in your sleep patterns: waking up often during the night, having trouble falling asleep, or wanting to sleep much of the time
- Changes in eating patterns: eating more or less than you used to, irrespective of hunger
- Difficulty concentrating or remembering things
- Fatigue and/or a lack of energy all the time
- Nervousness, irritability; inability to sit still
- Guilt: believing you "just can't do anything right" or that you are a burden to others
- Suicidal thoughts or attempts

Cognitive-behavioral therapy is based on the idea that your thoughts—and not external factors such as people or events—drive your behaviors and feelings. Therefore, you can change the way you think so that you will feel and behave better. Typically, individuals work with a therapist who helps them learn problem-solving skills that they can use to resolve stressful situations, as well as helps them identify their negative thought patterns and replace them with more positive ones (for example, helping patients realize that they *can* make positive changes in their lives that will reduce their risk of developing diabetic complications). (See the Suggested Reading List for resources detailing cognitive-behavioral therapy techniques.)

Unlike most other forms of psychotherapy, which typically involve years of sessions, cognitive-behavioral therapy is quick: the average number of sessions people need to reach their goals is sixteen. That's largely because cognitive-behavioral therapy is very interactive; you will learn specific techniques during your sessions, practice them during the week, and then report back to your therapist and discuss your experiences with the technique.

Margaret's Story

Margaret, a fifty-three-year-old school administrator, grew increasingly depressed in the year after she was diagnosed with type 2 diabetes. "I would go to work, go through the motions, and then go home and not feel like doing anything else," she says. "I used to be very active in a quilting group, and I loved to read and do gardening, but I found I didn't have the energy or the interest to do much of anything anymore." At the same time, Margaret wasn't eating right and often didn't bother to check her blood glucose levels. When she did take the time, she grew even more depressed with the results. Margaret's oldest daughter, Cynthia, was worried and convinced her mother to go to her doctor and get a referral to a therapist.

"I admit I didn't want to go originally, but then I was pleasantly surprised," says Margaret. "The therapist had me doing all kinds of assignments. She really made me work! One thing I had to do was write down every time I had a negative thought or expressed a negative comment, and then counter that negative event with a positive thought and write that down, too. One thing this exercise did was show me just how negative I was! During the first few days of doing the assignment, I was writing a lot. Then as time went on, I started to catch myself before expressing something negative and turn it into something positive. It sounded like such a silly exercise at first, but it was really very effective." Within a few months of starting her cognitive-behavioral sessions, Margaret had improved her diet, was monitoring her glucose levels regularly, and had returned to the hobbies she loved.

Cognitive-Behavioral Therapy Research

At Washington University School of Medicine in St. Louis, researchers wanted to find out whether diabetics who also had major depression would benefit from cognitive-behavioral therapy. A total of fifty-one patients were assigned to receive either ten weeks of individual cognitive-behavioral therapy (CBT) or no specific treatment. At the end of the study, 85 percent of the treated patients were in remission from depression, compared with 27 percent of the control patients. Six months later, the numbers were 70 percent and 33 percent, respectively. Furthermore, mean Hb A_{1c} levels were significantly better in the CBT group than in the control group (9.5 percent compared with 10.9 percent).

In another study, 240 depressed patients were treated with either antidepressants (paroxetine [Paxil] plus one other as needed), placebo, or cognitive-behavioral therapy for sixteen weeks. At the end of the study, 58 percent of patients in both the drug group and the therapy group responded to treatment, showing that drugs and therapy were equally effective. A follow-up study was then done with 104 of the patients who had responded to treatment. In this case, the patients stopped treatment—either CBT or medication—and were followed up with to see if the symptoms of major depression returned. The investigators found that patients who stopped CBT were less likely to relapse than those who stopped medication (31 percent relapse rate compared with 76 percent). More and more studies point to the effectiveness of cognitive-behavioral therapy in treating depression.

Other Nondrug Treatments for Diabetes Patients with Depression

While cognitive-behavioral therapy is effective in treating depression in people with diabetes, it is not the only effective nondrug approach for treating depression. Varying levels of success have been found with other interventions, including nutraceuticals (such as Saint-John's-wort, L-tryptophan, *Ginkgo biloba*), light therapy, exercise, stress-management techniques (covered in this chapter), prayer/spiritual guidance, and various mind-body therapies (for example, guided visualization, self-hypnosis, biofeedback). Please see the Suggested Reading List for resources that explore these other strategies for treating depression.

Drug Treatment for Diabetes Patients with Depression

As a treatment option, antidepressants or other drugs used to treat depression can be helpful, preferably as a short-term (less than six months) measure (see "Drugs Used to Treat Major or Clinical Depression," page 184). Most antidepressants work by helping make certain natural chemicals called neurotransmitters (serotonin, norepinephrine) more accessible to the brain. Neurotransmitters are necessary for normal brain function as well as the control of mood.

Some people find that taking an antidepressant during the first few months of therapy is just the extra lift they need to get them back on track, and then they stop the medication. This was the strategy Rosemary used to help beat her clinical depression.

"I had type 2 diabetes; I was overweight and depressed," says

DRUGS USED TO TREAT MAJOR OR CLINICAL DEPRESSION

Antidepressants:

- Selective serotonin reuptake inhibitors (SSRIs). These drugs usually produce fewer adverse effects than tricyclic drugs (see below) but are associated with gastrointestinal problems, sleep disturbances, and difficulties with sexual function and desire. Examples include citalopram (Celexa), escitalopram (Lexapro), fluoxetine (Prozac), paroxetine (Paxil), and sertraline (Zoloft).
- Tricyclics. These are widely used but cause bothersome side effects. Examples of drugs in this class include doxepin (Adapin, Sinequan), imipramine (Tofranil), desipramine (Norpramin), nortriptyline (Pamelor), and protriptyline (Vivactil).
- Monoamine oxidase (MAO) inhibitors. These old technology antidepressants are associated with a high risk of side effects and are not commonly used.
- Other antidepressants. Various other medications that are not chemically related fall into this category and include bupropion (Wellbutrin), maprotiline (Ludiomil), and trazodone (Desyrel).

Antianxiety medications: on occasion, an antianxiety drug is given along with an antidepressant early in the treatment of the condition. Alprazolam (Xanax), clonazepam (Klonopin), and lorazepam (Ativan) are a few of the drugs in this group. Side effects include drowsiness, loss of coordination, fatigue, and confusion.

the forty-five-year-old claims adjuster. "My doctor had given me an exercise program, but I didn't follow it. I just felt like it wasn't going to work anyway. Being overweight runs in my family." Rosemary's doctor referred her to a psychologist and also prescribed an antidepressant. After two months, Rosemary had joined a women's exercise group that she was attending regularly and reported that her mood was "100 percent better." Her doctor gradually took her off the antidepressant, and she says her exercise group "is my new drug. I've lost some weight, and I'm feeling much better. I'm glad to be off the antidepressant, and now my goal is to reduce my oral diabetic medication as well!"

Some diabetic patients who are treated for depression later find they can not only stop the antidepressant but also reduce or eliminate any oral diabetic medication they are taking. Like Rosemary, however, you must work with your doctor when adding and/or eliminating any type of medications for depression, diabetes, or any other conditions you are treating.

In a placebo-controlled, double-blind study conducted at the Washington University School of Medicine in St. Louis, researchers studied sixty people with diabetes who also had major depressive disorder. At the end of the eight-week study, those who had taken fluoxetine (Prozac) had significant improvement in both depression and blood sugar levels when compared with controls. Blood glucose levels improved because the drug reduced the body's response to the stress hormone cortisol, which the body releases during stressful situations. In a more recent study at the same university, bupropion (Wellbutrin) also was helpful in improving glucose control in a group of diabetes patients with major depression.

STRESS AND DIABETES

Richard Surwit, Ph.D., one of the foremost researchers of diabetes, metabolism, and stress, has been studying the relationship between stress hormones and blood glucose for more than twenty years, and he states with confidence that "stress does indeed raise blood sugar levels." He goes on to emphasize that even in people at risk for or who have prediabetes, "psychological factors may work to lower insulin secretion and raise blood sugar." It just so happens that the hormones psychologists call stress hormones are the same ones that can significantly impact blood glucose levels, and that these hormones (e.g., cortisol, epinephrine [also known as adrenaline], norepinephrine, and growth hormone) can have a serious negative impact on glucose metabolism unless they are controlled. Fortunately, simple stress-management techniques can be very successful at controlling hormone and glucose levels in people with diabetes when they are practiced regularly.

Acknowledging and Addressing Stress

First, let us be clear that the stress-management techniques we discuss in this chapter are not a substitute for diet, exercise, supplements, and/or medications. They are, however, scientifically proven complementary methods that, if practiced regularly, can impact your mental health and behaviors that lead to proactive, aggressive disease management.

The first step toward reaping the benefits of any stress-management techniques is to identify and acknowledge the presence of stress in your life. For many people, chronic stress has become "natural," and they don't even admit it's a problem. Lisa, for example, is a forty-one-year-old single working mother of two teenagers who has type 2 diabetes. Her children participate in after-school sporting events, which she often tries to attend after work, and she typically brings work home with her as well. Since her mother was diagnosed with cancer last year, she has spent much of her spare time helping with her care in a nearby town. To her credit, Lisa tries very hard to eat right and does monitor her glucose levels daily, but her doctor prescribed oral antidiabetes drugs for her when she consistently failed to keep her glucose levels within a reasonable range. She complains that she is always fatigued and that she has trouble sleeping.

Lisa was in a state of chronic stress, yet it wasn't until a diabetes educator talked with her and pointed it out that she thought about it. "I guess I knew at some level that I was overly stressed, but I was just too busy to even think about it, much less do anything about it."

For Lisa, a stress-management program that included daily progressive muscle relaxation practice was a turning point in her life and in how she managed her diabetes. "Within a few weeks of practicing progressive relaxation, I noticed results," she says. "My blood glucose levels improved, and I was starting to sleep better. After a month, my doctor reduced my medication by half, and after three months, I stopped taking it completely. I was so impressed with progressive relaxation that I taught it to my mother, and it's helping her too."

The Toll of Chronic Stress on Blood Glucose

Stress triggers the fight-or-flight response, an evolutionary adaptation that helped our ancestors to mobilize the stress hormones adrenaline and cortisol when fighting the wooly mammoth and the cave bear, but this response is maladaptive in modern society. The fight-or-flight response involves a host of bodily changes triggered by a surge in adrenaline and cortisol levels that impact blood pressure, breathing rate, muscle tension, and heart rate, as well as a slowdown in the activity of the gastrointestinal tract (intestines, stomach). Your body also increases blood sugar levels so you will have the energy to "escape" your dangerous situation.

If you have diabetes, and if your lifestyle is such that you are in a state of chronic or fairly constant stress, stress hormone levels can remain abnormally high, adding to your metabolic dysfunction, raising blood pressure, elevating cholesterol and triglyceride levels, and damaging your immune system.

Why Relaxation Techniques Help

Regardless of which relaxation technique you choose—meditation, yoga, tai chi, deep breathing, progressive relaxation—they all work in the same basic way. Focused relaxation thwarts the fight-or-flight response; it reduces the levels of stress hormones in your blood, which in turn allows all the bodily functions that were placed on red alert to return to normal.

CHOOSING A STRESS-MANAGEMENT TECHNIQUE

There are many different types of stress-reduction techniques, and some of them have undergone scientific scrutiny to determine whether they can effectively improve blood glucose levels and other factors associated with diabetes and metabolic syndrome. We look at three techniques that have proven records of success—progressive muscle relaxation, yoga and mindfulness meditation—and explain how you can include them in your life.

Progressive Muscle Relaxation

Progressive muscle relaxation is a stress-management technique that was developed by the physician Edmund Jacobson in the 1920s. It is a remarkably simple yet effective technique for reducing and even eliminating muscle tension, anxiety, and stress.

No special props are required; all you need is about ten to fifteen minutes of uninterrupted time to practice the technique, which involves voluntarily and systematically tensing and then relaxing the muscles in your body.

We suggest you record the following instructions for progressive relaxation by reading them slowly and leaving a fifteen-second pause between each step. Keep in mind that this exercise is about muscle discernment as well as relaxation. The first few times you do the exercise, you may have some difficulty zeroing in on specific muscles. This is normal; just relax and do the best you can, and soon it will become second nature.

- Lie down in a comfortable position, and close your eyes. Breathe slowly and easily.
- Focus on your left foot. Tense the muscles in your foot, and hold for eight seconds. Release the tension, and relax for fifteen seconds.
- Focus on your right foot. Tense the muscles in your foot, and hold for eight seconds. Release the tension, and relax for fifteen seconds.
- Focus on your lower left leg and foot. Tense the muscles, and hold for eight seconds. Release the tension, and relax for fifteen seconds.
- Focus on your lower right leg and foot. Tense the muscles, and hold for eight seconds. Release the tension, and relax for fifteen seconds.
- Focus on your entire left leg. Tense the muscles, and hold for eight seconds. Release the tension, and relax for fifteen seconds.
- Focus on your entire right leg. Tense the muscles, and hold for eight seconds. Release the tension, and relax for fifteen seconds.
- Focus on your buttocks. Tense the muscles, and hold for

eight seconds. Release the tension, and relax for fifteen seconds.

- Focus on your abdomen. Tense the muscles, and hold for eight seconds. Release the tension, and relax for fifteen seconds.
- Focus on your chest. Tense the muscles, and hold for eight seconds. Release the tension, and relax for fifteen seconds.
- Focus on your left hand. Make a tight fist, and hold for eight seconds. Release your fist, and relax for fifteen seconds.
- Focus on your right hand. Make a tight fist, and hold for eight seconds. Release your fist, and relax for fifteen seconds.
- Focus on your entire left arm. Tense the muscles, and hold for eight seconds. Release the tension, and relax for fifteen seconds.
- Focus on your entire right arm. Tense the muscles, and hold for eight seconds. Release the tension, and relax for fifteen seconds.
- Focus on your shoulders and neck. Tense the muscles, and hold for eight seconds. Release the tension, and relax for fifteen seconds.
- Focus on your face. Scrunch your face, and hold for eight seconds. Release the tension, and relax for fifteen seconds.
- Mentally scan your entire body, and note any area that still feels tense. Focus on that area, tense the muscles, and hold for eight seconds. Release the tension, and relax for fifteen seconds.
- When you are done, take several slow, deep breaths, and open your eyes.

The beneficial impact of progressive muscle relaxation on glucose levels and Hb A_{1c} levels has been demonstrated in various studies. A study published in 1983 was one of the first to show that this relaxation technique could significantly improve glucose tolerance. Dr. Surwit and his colleagues conducted a yearlong study completed by seventy-two patients with type 2 diabetes. The investigators found that compared with controls, patients who practiced stress-management skills (progressive muscle relaxation, breathing therapy, imagery) had a 0.5 percent reduction in Hb A_{1c} levels, which is associated with a significant reduction in the risk of microvascular complications, such as retinopathy. However, the reduction in Hb A_{1c} was 1 percent or greater in 32 percent of the treated patients, compared with only 12 percent of the controls.

Yoga

In recent years, yoga has shed its "mystical" or "new-age" label and become a mainstream practice across the United States. This is fortunate, because yoga has proven to be a safe and effective way to reduce stress and improve symptoms associated with serious medical conditions, such as diabetes, hypertension, and heart disease.

Although there are many different types of yoga, they all share the same central goal: to unite the body, mind, and spirit through the practice of physical movements and postures synchronized with breathing and focused awareness. The form most commonly practiced in the United States is hatha yoga, which is relatively slow paced and the form most suitable for beginners. Hatha yoga focuses on easy stretching and holding poses while integrating breathing into each movement. Iyengar yoga, a form of hatha, incorporates similar poses but focuses more on holding poses longer, which builds balance and strength. Both forms of yoga can significantly reduce stress and promote total body relaxation.

Evidence that yoga promotes relaxation and reduces stress has been measured scientifically. Researchers at Boston University School of Medicine and McLean Hospital in Belmont, Massachusetts, measured the levels of gamma-aminobutyric acid (GABA; a chemical involved in mood) in the brains of people after they practiced yoga and compared those levels with people who spent the same time reading. Those who practiced yoga had a 27 percent increase in GABA, which is similar to the response seen in people who take antidepressants. The readers did not experience an increase in GABA.

Other studies showed that people with type 2 diabetes who practiced yoga significantly reduced their fasting blood glucose levels, as well as their Hb A_{1c} levels, heart rate, and blood pressure, while also improving nerve function, which is important in preventing neuropathy. When researchers in Stockholm compared cognitive-behavioral therapy with yoga in volunteers during a four-month period, they found that all the participants experienced similar improvements in blood pressure, heart rate, quality of life, and stress reduction, which means either approach may help you in your stress-reduction efforts.

One review brought together the results of seventy studies that looked at the effects of yoga on cardiovascular disease (CVD) and CVD risk associated with insulin resistance. The investigators found that, overall, yoga may improve many risks associated with diabetes, including oxidative stress, insulin sensitivity, lipid levels, blood pressure, and glucose tolerance.

Yoga classes and instructions are widely available and offered by schools, private yoga instructors, community centers, senior centers, and fitness centers. Many offer free introductory sessions or even entire courses for little or no cost. Yoga also can be learned from tapes, DVDs, and books, although we recommend participating in individual or group yoga sessions at least in the beginning so you can learn the basics with a professional instructor. As always, talk to your doctor before beginning any new exercise program.

Mindfulness Meditation

More and more, meditation is gaining acceptance as an effective stress-management technique and is increasingly being recommended by enlightened (no pun intended) mainstream physicians. The benefits are many, and the downsides are virtually nonexistent. Once learned, meditation can be done anywhere and at any time you can set aside a few uninterrupted minutes. There is no cost, there are no side effects, and there are many different ways to do it; you choose the technique(s) that work best for you.

One reason for meditation's elevation in the eyes of mainstream medicine is that there's scientific research pointing to its effectiveness. In a study of more than ninety women with fibromyalgia, for example, those who underwent eight weekly sessions of mindfulness meditation (which we explain below) had a significant improvement in depressive symptoms when compared with women who did not meditate. Among older depressed adults, mindfulness meditation has been successful in alleviating depression.

Mindfulness meditation is one of the most common meditation approaches practiced in the United States. There are many books and tapes on how to practice mindfulness (see the Suggested Reading List), and with practice, preferably daily, you can have a significant positive impact on your glucose levels.

Mindfulness meditation is the practice of focusing your awareness on each moment; that is, your goal is to live each moment fully, which includes learning to accept and live with diabetes more completely. To get ready to meditate, find a place where you will not be interrupted for at least ten or fifteen minutes. Sit on a chair or on the floor with your back straight, or lie down. Once you learn mindfulness meditation, you may find yourself doing it while standing in line at the grocery store; some people become very good at practicing mindfulness just about anywhere.

Begin each session by taking a few slow, deep breaths and closing your eyes. Then focus on your breathing. You will likely become distracted by random thoughts, sounds in your environment, an itch or ache, or perhaps even odors. Mindfulness is about treating these distractions as though you were an objective observer, watching or being mindful of the distraction but letting it go by without allowing it to upset or affect you. In this way, you stay in the moment and maintain calm and harmony.

Meditation not only improves your ability to handle stress; it also lowers blood pressure, reduces heart rate, and improves mood. It's a stress-management tool that can be used by just about anyone.

PANIC, ANXIETY, AND DIABETES

According to the National Institute of Mental Health, about six million American adults have panic disorder, which is characterized by episodes involving overwhelming fear or anxiety, rapid heartbeat and/or breathing, trembling, profuse sweating, and feeling like you are going to die. Panic attacks occur twice as often in women as in men and are often accompanied by other serious conditions, including depression.

People with diabetes who experience repeated panic attacks are more likely to suffer severe health complications and are less likely to properly manage their disease, according to researchers in Seattle. They arrived at these findings when they studied

4,385 patients with diabetes, and 193 of them reported having panic attacks that caused them to change their behavior. Compared with diabetics who did not have panic attacks, those with panic disorder had a higher average Hb A_{1c} level (8.1 percent versus 7.7 percent) and more diabetes complications.

If you experience panic attacks or episodes of high anxiety, it is critical that you talk to your physician about treatment. Recognition and treatment of panic disorder and other psychological problems can go a long way toward improving your quality of life.

THE VALUE OF SUPPORT

The best diet, exercise plan, supplement program, glucose monitoring, stress management, and pharmaceutical treatment plan in the world won't do you a bit of good unless you implement them and maintain consistency with your program. Results of the Diabetes Prevention Program showed that ongoing education and support significantly reduced the risk of developing diabetes in people of all ages. In this program, participants who received ongoing counseling on diet, exercise, and behavior modification reduced their risk of developing diabetes by 58 percent, and in those aged sixty and older, the reduction in risk was 71 percent. The bottom line was that there was more than 100 percent increased relative risk of developing diabetes every year in those patients who did not receive education and ongoing support versus those who did.

Types of Support

External support comes in many forms. It may include help from professionals such as diabetes educators, health professionals who give talks in the community, professional societies like the American Diabetes Association (ADA), independent health and wellness organizations like Life Extension, and local experts involved with in-hospital or community-based diabetes self-management programs. More informal support may come from self-help groups and/or online support groups, and don't forget the invaluable moral support you can get from understanding and empathetic friends and family members. It's to your advantage to tap into all the support mechanisms you need to get a handle on your health. At the same time, you should always carefully weigh the information and advice you receive from any source, especially online support and self-help groups, no matter how well meaning the individual or group offering the information may be. Although people with prediabetes, metabolic syndrome, or diabetes share many characteristics, each person also has his or her own personal medical profile. An individualized approach is always best.

Diabetes Self-Management Education Programs

Diabetes self-management education programs are available throughout the United States, with dozens of programs in every state. The majority are offered by hospitals and health-care centers and are recognized by the American Diabetes Association. Depending on the facility, the program can include classes, support groups, and/or counseling services on all aspects of diabetes management, from basic information about the disease to meal planning, stress management, traveling with diabetes, weight management, effects of medication, glucose monitoring assistance, pregnancy and diabetes, and exercise plans. Professionals typically involved in such programs include dietitians, diabetes education nurses, exercise physiologists, and/or physicians. Most insurance plans cover the cost of these programs.

The American Diabetes Association

The American Diabetes Association (ADA) is a national non-profit organization that provides a variety of support services. The main Web site (www.diabetes.org), for example, has links to help you find a chapter of the ADA in your area, at which you can participate in activities, volunteer for events, and meet other people who have diabetes. The ADA main Web site also offers a link to various message boards that cover such topics as diet, exercise, diabetes in children, being newly diagnosed, and gestational diabetes.

National Diabetes Education Program

The National Diabetes Education Program is federally funded and is sponsored by the Centers for Disease Control and Prevention and the U.S. Department of Health and Human Services' National Institutes of Health. Each state has its own programs, information about which you can access at www.cdc.gov/diabetes/states/index.htm. The purpose of these programs is to provide information and services to individuals and groups to reduce the risks and complications associated with diabetes.

Self-Help and Support Groups

Both real and virtual (online) self-help and support groups can be a lifeline for people who, for whatever reason, are unable to access other diabetes services or groups or who want to take advantage of these groups in addition to other services. Gayle says she looks forward to sharing her thoughts and ideas with other type 2 diabetics in an online support group.

"I was diagnosed with diabetes just six months ago," says the thirty-eight-year-old advertising executive, "and I talked with a counselor at a diabetes self-management meeting right after

I was diagnosed. But I live pretty far from the city, and I don't like to drive into the city at night, so I can't attend any of the programs they sometimes run there. When I found some of the message boards and online support groups, I was really excited. I use three or four of them and have made some friends who have really helped me feel much less alone. I use it like a buddy system, plus we even exchange recipes."

Self-help and other groups can provide emotional support; empower and motivate you to make positive changes in your diet, exercise, and other lifestyle habits; and be a source of new coping strategies and skills. Some of these groups are led or monitored by health-care professionals, while others are run by laypeople. The caveats that go along with participating in such groups are (1) do not reveal personal information that will allow individuals to identify where you live or work; (2) talk to your health-care practitioner before you act on any suggestions or recommendations offered by group members; and (3) if you make plans to meet anyone or attend a group meeting that you learned about online, meet in a busy public place and/or bring a friend with you.

THE BOTTOM LINE

The prevention or treatment of diabetes can be greatly enhanced if you incorporate strategies to reduce stress and improve your mood. You can do both using little or no medication. Participation in diabetes education programs, as well as guidance from peers and/or health professionals, have been proven to be invaluable in keeping people with diabetes on track in their pursuit of health and well-being. We strongly encourage you to take advantage of educational and/or supportive diabetes programs or groups.

Chapter 10

A Pharmacologic Approach

Pharmaceutical drugs are powerful tools in the battle against diabetes and diabetes-related complications. However, the best medicine is prevention. Ideally, our goal is to use all the tools previously discussed to avoid diabetes altogether.

In my prior experience within the pharmaceutical industry, I had the opportunity to work with great medical scientists, terrific researchers, and dedicated clinical trial coordinators during global drug development programs for metabolic disease. During my tenure in the pharmaceutical industry, I learned many things. One key lesson is that pharmaceutical medications are tools, and like any tool, they can be very useful in the right situation, but one tool can't handle every task.

Because the majority of people with type 2 diabetes take at least one prescription medication, a question comes to mind: how well is conventional drug treatment serving their needs?

A 2006 study published in the journal *Diabetes Research and*

Clinical Practice sheds light on the question—and the answers. The investigators evaluated 532 patients from the National Health and Nutrition Examination Survey 2001–2002 who had diabetes to see how effective their antihypertensive, antidiabetes, and anticholesterol medications were in controlling cardiovascular risk factors. Those factors included blood pressure, lipids, and hemoglobin A_{1c} levels. Overall, 50.2 percent of the participants did not reach their goal value for Hb A_{1c}, 64.6 percent did not reach their LDL cholesterol goal, 52.3 percent missed their HDL cholesterol goal, 48.6 percent failed to reach their triglyceride goal, and 53 percent had elevated blood pressure. Only 12.7 percent of women and 5.3 percent of men had reached their goal values for Hb A_{1c}, blood pressure, and LDL simultaneously.

These results raise some provocative questions. For example, do diabetes patients take their medications faithfully? Do the medications not work well?

In fact, drugs are commonly thought to be "magic bullets" for any disease, not just diabetes. This type of thinking is a major mistake in diabetes. In fact, drugs work best when they are part of a comprehensive program that includes diet, nutrition, exercise, behavioral changes, and so on. The focus of our program remains the same—we need to address and correct core causes of diabetes and metabolic disease (e.g., the interrelated factors of insulin resistance and beta-cell dysfunction) and diabetes-related complications (e.g., the interrelated factors of glycation, oxidative stress, and inflammation) in order to optimally attack the problem.

THE MEDICINE CABINET

Several major classes of oral antidiabetes drugs as well as insulin itself are used in the treatment of hyperglycemia (high blood sugar). There are also drugs used to treat diabetes-associated conditions, such as high blood pressure, high cholesterol, and cardiovascular concerns.

Currently, there are innovative new classes of drugs that target beta-cell dysfunction, a core cause of metabolic disease and type 2 diabetes. In fact, these drugs represent the most important advance in the drug treatment of diabetes in the past few years. These new drugs target incretins (which we explain below) and include glucagon-like peptide and dipeptidyl peptidase inhibitors.

INCRETIN MIMETICS AND DIPEPTIDYL PEPTIDASE INHIBITORS

Although you may be tempted to skip this section because the drug categories appear esoteric and/or arcane, we urge you to read and become knowledgeable about these drugs so that you can become fully involved in treatment decisions made with your physician. These new, innovative drugs represent the most significant breakthrough in diabetes treatment options, in our opinion, in many years, because they target a fundamental cause of diabetes—beta-cell function.

In an effort to avoid confusion, let us explain that within the broader class of drugs known as incretins is a subclass called dipeptidyl peptidase (DPP-4) inhibitors, so we will discuss them together. Incretin mimetics are aptly named because they mimic the glucose-lowering actions of natural hormones in the body called incretins. The key incretin is glucagon-like peptide GLP-1. This gut-derived hormone protects beta cells, stimulates the secretion of insulin, inhibits the secretion of glucagon, and can also help you lose weight by enhancing satiety (the sensation of feeling satisfied from eating). As of the time of this writing, the sole drug in the incretin mimetic class is exenatide.

DIABETES MEDICATIONS

Sulfonylureas: *First generation:* chlorpropamide (Diabinese), tolazamide (Tolinase), and tolbutamide (Orinase); *second generation:* glipizide (Glucotrol) and glyburide (Diabeta, Glynase, Micronase); *third generation:* glimepiride (Amaryl)

Meglitinides: nateglinide (Starlix) and repaglinide (Prandin)

Biguanide: metformin (Glucophage, Glucophage XR)

Alpha-glucosidase inhibitors: acarbose (Precose), miglitol (Glyset)

Thiazolidinediones (TZDs): rosiglitazone (Avandia), pioglitazone (Actos)

Insulins: aspart (NovoLog), lispro (Humalog), regular (Humulin R, Novolin R), intermediate (Humulin N, Novolin N), glargine (Lantus), ultralente (Humulin U), lente (Humulin L), glulisine (Apidra), plus combination products: Humulin 70/30, Humulin 50/50, Novolin 70/30, among others

Combinations: combination medications include Avandaryl (rosiglitazone plus glimepiride) and Avandamet (rosiglitazone plus metformin)

Incretins (glucagon-like peptide [GLP-1] mimetics and dipeptidyl peptidase [DPP-4] inhibitors): exenatide (Byetta), sitagliptin (Januvia). Another DPP-4 inhibitor is slated for approval at the time of this writing, tentatively called Galvus.

Exenatide got its start in monsters—Gila monsters, that is. The drug was originally isolated from the salivary glands of the North American lizard known as the Gila monster. This lizard eats large meals very infrequently and secretes exendin-4, a substance that causes the pancreas to "wake up" and secrete insulin, a characteristic that makes it a candidate for diabetes treatment. The amazing promise with exenatide—unlike every other antidiabetes drug on the market before this drug was FDA-approved—is that it may help *regenerate* beta cells. There is tantalizing evidence from experimental studies that this may, in fact, be true, but more research needs to occur to confirm this potential breakthrough. GLP-1–directed therapies like ex-enatide also slow the emptying of the stomach, which enhances satiety and suppresses further food intake, and inhibits the overproduction of glucose by the liver. All these critical proper-ties make exenatide an important addition to the prescription drug arsenal we have on hand to fight diabetes.

Another major, previously unknown attribute of exenatide and oral DPP-4 inhibitors is that incretins enhance insulin secretion in a glucose-dependent manner. Old-technology therapies like sulfonylureas promote insulin secretion in a glucose-independent fashion, which means they cause beta cells to secrete insulin regardless of what your blood sugar level is, be it 500 mg/dL or 50 mg/dL. New-technology drugs like exena-tide are glucose-dependent, which means they prompt the beta cells to secrete insulin only when blood sugar levels are high. Thus, exenatide will not cause already low blood sugar levels to fall even lower, to potentially dangerous levels.

The old-technology therapy can cause some problems. For example, if your blood sugar level is 50 mg/dL, sulfonylureas will continue to prompt the beta cell to secrete insulin. Since a blood sugar of 50 mg/dL is quite low, any additional decline re-sults in hypoglycemia (abnormally low blood sugar levels) and can lead to brain damage, seizures, and/or death.

HYPOGLYCEMIA UNAWARENESS: LITTLE DISCUSSED BUT POTENTIALLY DEADLY

The treatment for low blood sugar is simple—eat some carbohydrate.

However, a potentially deadly complication of long-term diabetes is hypoglycemia unawareness, a condition whereby patients are unable to sense the typical symptoms of low blood sugar—nausea, tremors, light-headedness, dizziness, anxiety, and heart palpitations. This condition can place patients at risk for extended exposure to very low blood sugar levels and can result in loss of consciousness, seizure, and even death.

Old-technology drugs like sulfonylureas that prompt insulin secretion in a glucose-independent fashion place patients at greater risk for hypoglycemia because they trigger insulin secretion without regard to blood sugar level.

The many benefits of exenatide are countered by a few downsides: it is injectable, and it can cause nausea (however, nausea almost always disappears within a short time after the beginning of treatment). Headache, vomiting, diarrhea, and nervousness may also occur.

The subclass of DPP-4 inhibitors had one FDA-approved member as of mid-2007, and another drug, called vildagliptin (Galvus), was expected to be approved by the end of the year, with three more drugs in this subclass also in development. The approved drug is sitagliptin (Januvia), which targets DPP-4, an enzyme that blocks the signals your body sends to balance high blood glucose levels. When a DPP-4 inhibitor blocks this enzyme, it prolongs the blood levels of GLP-1, which in turn causes the cascade of beneficial effects similar to the GLP-1 mimetic Byetta (exenatide).

Two of the experts who originally discovered the benefits of DPP-4 note that because drugs like sitagliptin stimulate beta-cell function, they will likely work best in people who have prediabetes, because these people still have enough beta cells that can be "urged" to prevent progression of the disease. Once people are diagnosed with diabetes, only about 50 percent of normal beta-cell function remains.

Studies of sitagliptin show that it can reduce Hb A_{1c} levels by nearly 3 percent in patients who start with high Hb A_{1c} levels, which is significantly better than other available drugs. Currently, investigators are looking at the effectiveness of a combination of sitagliptin and metformin. When taken alone, DPP-4 inhibitors may cause runny/stuffy nose, headache, diarrhea, and sore throat.

Sulfonylureas

As you can likely guess, we are not big believers in the use of sulfonylureas as beta cell–directed therapies for diabetes treatment. First introduced into the United States in 1955, sulfonylureas stimulate the beta cells to produce more insulin. As we mentioned in earlier chapters, hyperinsulinemia (high insulin levels) is common among people who have early-stage type 2 diabetes, and we believe that taking sulfonylureas, which act in a glucose-independent fashion (regardless of blood sugar level), places undue stress on the beta cells to produce insulin and may actually hasten *progression* of beta-cell burnout. In fact, this has been a nagging concern among diabetes experts for a number of years, but prior to the approval of GLP-1 and DPP-4 technologies, there were no new beta cell–directed drugs available. We have already noted that sulfonylureas are a frequent cause of hypoglycemia, especially when long-acting first-generation drugs from this drug class are used. Drugs in the second and third generation (less long acting) are less likely to cause low blood sugar. Studies also suggest that some of the sulfonylureas, including glyburide and tolbutamide, increase the risk of cardiac problems.

Meglitinides

Only two drugs are in this class, and both cause a rapid rise in insulin levels by stimulating the beta cells independent of blood sugar levels. The activity of meglitinides peaks in one hour and lasts only three hours, which means they work best when taken shortly before meals so they can address rising glucose levels after eating. A downside of the meglitinides, however, is that you must remember to take them before each meal. Side effects may include low blood sugar, nausea, vomiting, diarrhea, muscle aches, sore joints, headache, flu-like symptoms, and back pain.

Biguanide

Metformin is the only drug in this class, and it is also the most often prescribed antidiabetes drug on the market. This drug performs several functions, the most important of which is its ability to increase the body's sensitivity to insulin. It also inhibits the overproduction of glucose by the liver, helps with weight loss, improves endothelial function, and favorably affects cholesterol and triglyceride levels. When used alone, it rarely causes hypoglycemia (abnormally low blood glucose). The drug comes in two forms: regular, which can be taken before meals, and extended release, which can be taken once daily. It is often prescribed along with another insulin sensitizer drug class, thiazolidinediones.

Potential side effects include diarrhea, bloating, constipation, and heartburn. If you have congestive heart failure, kidney or liver disease, or if you drink an excessive amount of alcohol, you should not take metformin. Everyone who takes metformin should have their kidney function evaluated at least once a year, and blood levels of vitamin B_{12} and folic acid should be assessed regularly, as metformin use has occasionally been associated with a deficiency of these essential vitamins.

On very rare occasions, metformin has been linked to a condition called lactic acidosis, which is characterized by unusual fatigue or severe drowsiness, muscle pain, breathing difficulties, irregular or unusually slow heartbeat, and cold skin. The people most likely to develop these symptoms are those older than eighty who have not had their kidney and/or liver function evaluated; those who have liver or kidney disease, a serious infection, poor circulation, or dehydration; anyone who uses excessive amounts of alcohol; or those who have received an injectable iodinated contrast drug for a scanning or x-ray procedure.

Alpha-Glucosidase Inhibitors

The drugs in this class inhibit the digestion of carbohydrate, which in turn reduces your postprandial (after eating) blood glucose levels. Use of these drugs can help some people lose weight easier, and they can be used in combination with sulfonylureas, metformin, and/or insulin. Side effects, however, can be significant: flatulence occurs in up to 77 percent of patients, diarrhea affects up to one-third, and stomach pain is experienced by up to 21 percent.

Alpha-glucosidase inhibitors have not proven to be very effective in lowering Hb A_{1c} levels. These drugs should not be used by people who have limited kidney function or bowel disorders, nor should they be taken by nursing mothers.

Thiazolidinediones

Improved insulin sensitivity and reduced liver glucose levels are the goals of the drugs in this class. There is also evidence that they improve cholesterol levels and favor a beneficial redistribution of body fat (i.e., less abdominal fat and more peripheral body fat). The side effects of thiazolidinediones (TZDs) include fluid retention and liver toxicity. The latter complication requires that you have regular monitoring of your liver function.

Several significant warnings about TZDs emerged in 2007. In February of that year, the manufacturers of Avandia (rosiglitazone) reported that in their study of more than 4,300 patients with type 2 diabetes, significantly more women who took rosiglitazone experienced fractures of the foot, hand, or upper arm than did women who were taking metformin or glyburide. More research into this complication is ongoing, but results are not expected until 2009.

On May 21, 2007, the Food and Drug Administration issued a news release in which it stated that rosiglitazone was associated with an increased risk of heart attack and other heart-related conditions. The related article published in the *New England Journal of Medicine* reported that the risks were 43 percent for heart failure and 64 percent for death from cardiovascular causes.

Insulins

For people who have type 1 diabetes, insulin is a life-saving medication that must be taken every day. Our goal when working with people who have type 2 diabetes, however, is to use the comprehensive approach we have presented throughout this book to control beta-cell function and insulin sensitivity in an effort to reverse the course of the disease. Twenty-seven percent of people with type 2 diabetes currently use insulin, yet less than half of them are able to bring their Hb A_{1c} level below 7 percent. Insulin can be useful on a temporary basis if you have an acute illness, are undergoing surgery, or are pregnant.

The types and dosages of insulin you need will depend on your medical situation and lifestyle (dietary and exercise habits) and should be discussed with your physician. Currently there are seven types of insulin products available for people who have diabetes.

- Rapid-acting: begins working in five to twenty minutes and finishes in three to five hours
- Short-acting: begins in thirty minutes and works for five to eight hours. It is one of the two most commonly used types of insulin.
- Intermediate-acting: begins in one to three hours and works for sixteen to twenty-four hours. It is one of the two most commonly used types of insulin.
- Long-acting: begins in four to six hours and works for twenty-four to twenty-eight hours
- Very long acting: begins in one hour and works for twenty-four hours
- Premixed (combined short- and intermediate-acting): begins in thirty minutes and works for sixteen to twenty-four hours

The seventh type is inhaled insulin, which generally consists of a powdered formulation that you inhale into your lungs. Inhaled insulin is formulated in such a way as to optimize pulmonary (lung) delivery and absorption.

Inhaled insulin is not for everyone. If you have asthma, bronchitis, emphysema, or if you smoke or recently quit smoking (within six months), you should not use this drug. Because of possible damage to the lungs, you should have your lung function checked six months after starting to use inhalable insulin, and then every year thereafter. Furthermore, if you currently need injectable insulin, inhaled insulin can be used at mealtime, but not as a replacement for your longer-acting injections.

Although we are enthusiastic about the mealtime convenience of inhaled insulin, there remain residual, open-ended questions about the possible long-term effects this type of insulin delivery system may have on the lungs.

Diabetes Medication Combinations

Many people with diabetes are taking more than one antidiabetes medication or are taking one of the newer combination drugs. Sulfonylureas are sometimes taken along with metformin or TZDs for improved glycemic control, while TZDs are taken with metformin for improved glycemic control, insulin sensitivity, and beta-cell health.

Several name-brand combination drugs for treating type 2 diabetes are on the market. This is largely an attempt by the pharmaceutical companies to squeeze more patent life (and profit) out of expiring drugs.

HORMONE RESTORATION

For many aging men and women, hormone restoration has made dramatic, positive changes in their lives. Hormone restoration/replacement (estrogen, progesterone, and/or testosterone) in men and women must be evaluated carefully, with a full and careful assessment of the risks and benefits on an individual basis. In men, this includes a careful assessment of prostate cancer risk, and in women, a detailed risk/benefit evaluation with careful attention to hormone-responsive cancers of the breast and endometrium. It is essential that you work closely with a qualified, experienced doctor well versed in hormone replacement/restoration to maximize effectiveness and minimize risk.

All aging men should take the time to have their free and total testosterone, estradiol (a type of estrogen), and dihydrotestosterone (DHT; a testosterone derivative) levels checked. In fact, low levels of testosterone are associated with metabolic syndrome and type 2 diabetes. Up to one-third of men with type 2 diabetes have low levels of testosterone, which means they are at risk for loss of bone density and muscle tone, an increase in abdominal fat, and changes in mood and cognition, as well as reduced sex drive and erectile dysfunction.

For many aging men who are deficient in testosterone, replacement to an optimal level can make a dramatic difference. Studies show that testosterone replacement in aging men can result in improvement in their cardiovascular and diabetic risk factors, including blood glucose, cholesterol, blood pressure, insulin resistance, insulin sensitivity, and/or Hb A_{1c}. Replacement can also help with erectile dysfunction. A number of experimental studies show that the hormone testosterone can restore the ability to have an erection and the ability to respond to treatment with sildenafil (Viagra).

If you are a perimenopausal or postmenopausal woman, hormone replacement therapy (HRT) is a controversial topic. The 2003 published results of the Women's Health Initiative (WHI) study, which used conjugated equine estrogens and synthetic progestogens (progestins), showed mixed results and raised a great number of questions. The WHI study results included evidence of an increase in the risk for breast cancer and heart disease, yet reduced the risk of hip fractures and colorectal cancer. One reason for the results in the WHI trial is the use of synthetic progestogens rather than natural progesterone.

LOW TESTOSTERONE IS COMMON IN DIABETIC MEN

A study in the November 2004 issue of the *Journal of Clinical Endocrinology and Metabolism* revealed that one out of three diabetic men have low testosterone levels. Researchers at the University at Buffalo and Kaleida Health in Buffalo, New York, measured the serum testosterone and other associated hormone levels of 103 men who had type 2 diabetes. None of the men had previously been diagnosed with low testosterone levels. It was discovered that 33 percent of them had low levels of the hormone. Low levels of testosterone are associated with a number of adverse health conditions, including erectile dysfunction, loss of muscle tone, increased abdominal fat, low bone density, poor mood, and decreased cognitive function. We recommend that men with diabetes or prediabetes have their hormone levels checked, because of the relationship between low testosterone, abdominal obesity, and insulin resistance.

The overall evidence suggests that synthetic progestogens like medroxyprogesterone acetate (MPA) are inferior to natural progesterone. The risk of breast cancer associated with HRT in 54,548 postmenopausal women who had never taken any HRT was studied in the E3N-EPIC (National Education System-European Prospective Investigation into Cancer & Nutrition) study. HRT containing synthetic progestogens was associated with a 40 percent increase in the risk of breast cancer as opposed to no increase in risk with HRT that contained micronized progesterone.

When it comes to metabolic function, studies suggest that synthetic progestogens may worsen insulin sensitivity. There is also evidence that women of childbearing age who use contraceptives that contain synthetic progestogens may be at increased risk for gestational diabetes. A recent study showed that the risk was greater among women who took a higher-dose progestin compared with those who took a lower dose.

ANTIGLYCATION MEDICATIONS

Since glycation is a major theme of this book, we'll take a brief look at several drugs that directly target glycation. One of the drugs is aminoguanidine, a compound that blocks glycation-induced damage in experimental models of diabetic kidney disease (nephropathy) and diabetic eye disease (retinopathy). Aminoguanidine has also been shown to block glycation-induced diabetic vascular damage. However, there are side effects associated with the use of aminoguanidine, including the fact that it inhibits the synthesis of an important blood vessel–dilating molecule, nitric oxide, which makes taking it a cardiovascular risk.

A more familiar drug with antiglycation properties is aspirin. Aspirin inhibits the development of diabetic retinopathy, and a recent study showed that it can inhibit the formation of pentosidine, a glycation end product. Other drugs with antiglycation properties include angiotensin-converting enzyme (ACE) inhibitors. We'll discuss the antiglycation properties of ACE inhibitors in more detail when we discuss antihypertensive medications.

Two possible entries (drugs not yet approved by the FDA) in the antiglycation drug arena include pyridoxamine, a substance that has shown powerful antiglycation effects in experimental models of diabetic kidney disease, and ALT-946, a drug still in the development stage that appears to be a more potent inhibitor of glycation-induced damage than aminoguanidine but that has limited effects on nitric oxide production. You may see these drugs in the near future.

TREATING CARDIOVASCULAR RISKS

Although diet, nutraceuticals, and lifestyle strategies are critical interventions for supporting cardiovascular health, prediabetic and diabetic patients often need pharmacological medications to optimally treat cardiovascular problems like high blood pressure, high cholesterol, and/or high triglycerides.

Treating High Blood Pressure

If you have type 2 diabetes and your blood pressure is not well controlled (we recommend a blood pressure target of less than 125/75 mm Hg), does it matter which drug you take to bring your blood pressure down and help prevent cardiovascular disease?

This very question helped spur the ALLHAT (Antihypertensive and Lipid-Lowering Treatment to Prevent Heart Attack Trial), the largest hypertension clinical trial ever conducted, back in 2002. The experts looked at three different classes of medication for high blood pressure: a thiazide diuretic (chlorthalidone [Hygroton, Thalitone]), an ACE inhibitor (lisinopril [Zestril, Prinivil]), and a calcium channel–blocker (amlodipine [Norvasc]). The study concluded that the cheap and cost-effective diuretic chlorthalidone was superior to the other drug types when it came to preventing cardiovascular disease in hypertensive patients with prediabetes and diabetes. This finding was reaffirmed in a 2007 validation study of ALLHAT. Overall, when compared with the ACE inhibitor and calcium channel–blocker, the diuretic worked just as well for protecting against heart attack and improving survival.

There were a number of limitations with the ALLHAT study

design. Previous studies found that ACE inhibitors slowed the progression of kidney damage in diabetic patients with kidney disease. However, because ALLHAT did not collect urine samples to measure urine microalbuminuria, a comparison of kidney protection effectiveness for ACE inhibitors versus diuretics was not possible. An interesting component of ACE inhibitors also not considered in ALLHAT is that they protect against glycotoxin-induced damage.

In addition to the ALLHAT study, other research has shown that the ACE inhibitor ramipril (Tritace, Altace) significantly reduced the incidence of death (by 24 percent), stroke (33 percent), myocardial infarction (22 percent), cardiovascular death (37 percent), and nephropathy (24 percent) compared with placebo. Several studies indicate that ACE inhibitors help prevent diabetic complications, including atherosclerosis, by preventing glycotoxins from damaging the delicate endothelium of blood vessels. In the Heart Outcomes Prevention Evaluation (HOPE) study, for example, patients who were taking ramipril had significantly lower levels of glycotoxins than patients in the placebo group. In an experimental model of diabetes, two different ACE inhibitors were successful in reducing glycotoxin levels. Other studies have resulted in similar findings. Overall, the ability of ACE inhibitors to protect against glycotoxin damage, reduce blood pressure, and protect the kidneys makes these drugs very attractive treatment options for type 2 diabetes.

A cautionary note on the antihypertensive drug class known as beta-blockers: researchers who studied more than 143,000 nondiabetic patients who had high blood pressure showed that patients who took beta-blockers were much more likely to develop diabetes than patients who took ACE inhibitors or angiotensin-receptor blockers (ARBs). Calcium channel–blockers were in between: they were not as protective as ACE inhibitors or ARBs but more so than beta-blockers.

Treating High Cholesterol

Diabetics suffer heart attacks and strokes at a greatly increased rate compared with people without diabetes. People with diabetes almost always have high triglycerides, low good HDL, and high bad LDL levels, with a tendency to form small, dense, atherogenic (artery-clogging) LDL particles. Given that insulin resistance is a major cardiovascular disease risk factor, should all patients with insulin resistance and type 2 diabetes be taking a cholesterol-lowering statin drug regardless of their cholesterol level? To get an answer to this question, read on.

RECOMMENDED CHOLESTEROL GOALS AND SOME TREATMENT OPTIONS

Goals

LDL: < 100 mg/dL (< 70 mg/dL if you recently had a heart attack or acute coronary syndrome)
HDL: > 60 mg/dL for men and women
Triglycerides: < 100 mg/dL

Treatment Options

Statins: atorvastatin (Lipitor), fluvastatin (Lescol), lovastatin (Mevacor), pravastatin (Pravachol), rosuvastatin calcium (Crestor), simvastatin (Zocor)
Fibrates: bezafibrate (Bezalip), fenofibrate (Lofibra, TriCor), gemfibrozil (Lopid)
Nicotinic acid: niacin (over-the-counter), Niaspan (prescription)

Statins are the drugs most commonly prescribed to treat abnormal lipid levels, and specifically elevated LDL cholesterol, which typically is the main target of cholesterol therapy. Several major statin trials, including three large, older trials and three more recent studies, have included patients with diabetes. Unfortunately, the benefits (or lack of benefits) of statins for patients with type 2 diabetes are not clear from the results of these trials for various reasons, including study-design flaws, technical issues relating to statistics, and the small numbers of diabetic patients involved in some of the trials.

The best argument for the use of statins to reduce the risk of heart disease in diabetes can be seen in the results of the double-blind, placebo-controlled Collaborative Atorvastatin Diabetes Study (CARDS), in which more than 2,800 men and women participated. Daily treatment with a statin reduced major cardiovascular events by 37 percent compared with a placebo. Of great importance, the benefit to patients was observed independent of their LDL-cholesterol or triglyceride levels at the start of the study.

Based on the results of the CARDS study, we believe that patients with type 2 diabetes should strongly consider speaking with their physicians about taking a low-dose statin to reduce the risk of heart attack or other major cardiovascular event. We also believe that the lowest possible dose of statin should be used to achieve target cholesterol levels in diabetics and non-diabetics alike.

If you take a statin, we recommend that you supplement it with CoQ10. Statins deplete CoQ10 levels, and supplements help to minimize or avoid altogether many of the side effects associated with statins, including muscle pain and memory problems. In the vast majority of cases, CoQ10 supplementation dramatically reduces statin-induced side effects.

A potentially very dangerous but rare side effect associated with high doses of potent statin drugs is muscle damage called rhabdomyolysis. If you take statin drugs and experience severe muscle pain or weakness, contact your physician immediately.

Niacin is available as a supplement as well as in a prescription, sustained-release form. The prescription form is significantly more costly and not much better in terms of side-effect profile or tolerability.

There are three forms of niacin available: nicotinic acid, nicotinamide, and inositol hexaniacinate. Nicotinic acid can decrease triglycerides and raise HDL cholesterol, but this requires high doses (typically 1.5 to 3 g daily), which can cause flushing and liver toxicity. (As a general precaution, anyone who takes more than 2 g of niacin daily or more than 500 mg at the same time as statins should undergo periodic liver function tests.) Nicotinic acid may also worsen glycemic control.

Nicotinamide may be effective in supporting blood sugar levels and may prevent the development of diabetes in certain high-risk groups, although trial results so far have been mixed. Inositol hexaniacinate is less likely to cause flushing, but it does not have the potent lipid-regulating qualities of nicotinic acid.

THE BOTTOM LINE

Our goal is to provide a comprehensive, evidence-based strategy to prevent metabolic disease, or if you already have insulin resistance or type 2 diabetes, to reverse the course of the disease. Medications are tools that can help with this goal. We strongly advise you to speak with your doctor about the best tools and interventions to use in your case, based on your medical needs. We believe that some of the newer drugs on the market—the DPP-4 inhibitors and incretin mimetics—along with the older drug metformin, have interesting properties and characteristics that make them attractive options. Prevention, however, is still the best solution.

Chapter 11

Stories to Tell

LARRY'S STORY

Larry, a sixty-one-year-old physician living in Dallas, Texas, spends most of his days consulting with and advising individuals on how they can best optimize their health and the health of their loved ones. He is well versed in and has access to the latest nutritional supplements, prescription drugs, and various wellness strategies that are available.

When Larry uncovered his own case of type 2 diabetes in June 2005, he already knew a great deal about the dangers of glycation and glycotoxins and immediately adjusted his diet to minimize their damaging effects. In fact, he and his wife both dedicated themselves to "cleaning up" their eating habits by switching to poaching and steaming instead of grilling and frying and limiting their consumption of high-protein and high-fat foods. "Gloria does most of the cooking," says Larry, "so it only made sense for her to come on board with the adjustments as well. And it's really great for her, too. I don't want her to ever have to worry about having diabetes." Along with the dietary changes, Larry was taking the DPP-4 inhibitor sitagliptin (Januvia).

Larry's methods seemed to be paying off: he had excellent control of his blood glucose, reflected in his impressive 5.1 percent Hb A_{1c} results. Yet his serum cholesterol and lipid profile continued to be less than ideal, and he was not pleased. In April 2006, his HDL cholesterol was 47 mg/dL, and his baseline serum triglyceride level was 237 mg/dL. Although the HDL figure was not a great concern (less than 40 mg/dL is cause for concern in men), we always strive to raise this good cholesterol level. Larry's triglyceride level was significantly higher than the 150 mg/dL upper limit for normal, and this was his area of greatest worry.

Larry had a decision to make: introduce a statin drug into his daily routine or try a natural supplement. He reviewed the supplements that could help him change these figures and chose high-quality omega-3 fatty acids in the form of a fish oil, olive fruit, and sesame lignans proprietary product. After taking the fish oil supplement for five months, his triglyceride level dropped to 128 mg/dL and his HDL improved to 79 mg/dL, reflecting a remarkable 46 percent decrease in triglycerides and a 40 percent improvement in HDL. Larry continues to take the fish oil supplement and maintain good glucose control and an impressive Hb A_{1c} reading. And despite a family history of type 2 diabetes, Gloria maintains a healthy Hb A_{1c} herself, a fasting glucose level in the 80s, and believes their new eating habits are a "very big contributing factor" in her ability to steer clear of type 2 diabetes.

MELANIE AND BRAD'S STORY

It's typical of married couples to share many things in their lives—the same taste in music, a love of the outdoors, favorite foods, the same type of movies—but for some, the sharing extends to health issues. For Melanie and Brad, the shared issue is type 2 diabetes.

Both Melanie and Brad are in their middle thirties, and they both work full time, Melanie as a public relations manager and Brad as a math professor at a junior college. Brad was first diagnosed with type 2 diabetes in late 2005 after undergoing a fasting glucose test that was part of the physical required by the college. Although Brad was moderately overweight, he had no known family history of diabetes, as he had been adopted and did not know his birth parents. Because his fasting glucose level was greater than 150 mg/dL and his postmeal levels were typically near 300 mg/dL, his doctor immediately wrote a prescription for metformin (Glucophage) and glyburide (Micronase).

A few months later Melanie made her appointment for a fasting blood glucose test. Melanie is slightly overweight and has a family history of type 2 diabetes, so she knew she should have her blood glucose checked regularly. She had neglected to do so for several years, however, and Brad's diagnosis prompted her to make the appointment. In early 2006 Melanie's doctor told her that her fasting glucose level was 124 mg/dL and that she was at risk for developing type 2 diabetes. He wrote her a prescription for the antidiabetes drug metformin (Glucophage) and arranged for her to have a session with a diabetes education counselor, who showed her how to use a glucose monitor and talked about diet. Melanie began to carefully track her blood glucose levels every day.

During the first few months on metformin, Melanie's fasting blood glucose readings averaged 129 mg/dL, while her postmeal blood glucose readings averaged 148 mg/dL. Melanie ranked this range as "not good enough," as she was concerned that given her family history, she needed to be more aggressive about avoiding diabetes. After talking with her doctor, she began taking a daily supplement of cinnamon extract standardized for water-soluble polyphenols. After taking the cinnamon supplement for only three months, her fasting blood glucose levels improved to an average of 98 mg/dL, and her postprandial levels averaged 118 mg/dL. Impressed, she then added chromium, coffee berry extract, and benfotiamine to her daily regimen, and her blood sugar levels improved so much over the next few months that her doctor told her she could stop taking metformin. She continues to be drug-free, is taking all four supplements, and her blood glucose levels remain good: 90 mg/dL average for fasting levels and 114 mg/dL average after meals.

At first, Brad was skeptical about his wife's "experimenting" with herbal supplements. When she began to get good results, however, he decided it was time to ask his doctor about adding supplements to his drug therapy, which was still leaving him with blood glucose levels ranging from 200 to 260 mg/dL. Brad added coffee berry extract, chromium, and water-soluble cinnamon extract to his daily routine, and within three months, his blood glucose levels had declined significantly; they are now consistently lower than 200 mg/dL and average 160 mg/dL.

FRANK'S STORY

Early in 2006, Frank, a fifty-seven-year-old retired police officer who now runs a security company out of his home, noticed that he was feeling very tired. He also found that he was thirsty much of the time for no apparent reason, that his vision was frequently blurry, and that his fingers would often become numb.

The combination of symptoms concerned him, so he made an appointment with his family doctor. His physical examination and blood profile showed a clear picture of diabetes:

- Fasting glucose, 185 mg/dL
- Blood pressure, 150/80 mm Hg
- Hemoglobin A_{1c}, 13.2 percent
- Total cholesterol, 220 mg/dL
- HDL, 25 mg/dL
- Triglycerides, 390 mg/dL

Frank was also overweight, carrying 250 pounds on his 5-foot, 10-inch frame. His family history also raised some red flags. His one older sister, Margaret, had been diagnosed with diabetes at age fifty-five, while his mother had died of a heart attack at age sixty-two. "I don't know whether my mother had diabetes," says Frank, "but she was overweight and had high blood pressure. My father died in an automobile accident at age fifty-nine, and I don't know about his medical history except that he, too, was overweight."

Frank's physician started him on sitagliptin (Januvia), 100 mg daily. He also prescribed alpha-lipoic acid, 600 mg daily, because of the neuropathy and family history of heart disease and diabetes. Frank's diet needed some major overhauling, so his physician arranged for him to have several sessions with a diabetes educator, as well as get information on an antiglycation eating program. Frank was also encouraged to include his wife in the sessions and for her to read and ask questions about the new eating program for her husband.

To facilitate weight loss, Frank started an aggressive walking program. Although he considered the modified Tabata approach as presented in chapter 7, for the first three months he decided to see how much weight he could lose with a combination of new eating habits and walking. His exercise consisted of ten minutes of stretching, followed by fifteen minutes of brisk walking (which he gradually increased to forty minutes over a three-month period), and then another five minutes of stretching. Frank followed this routine four days per week.

At the end of three months, Frank's Hb A_{1c} was 7.9 percent, he had lost 22 pounds, and his fasting glucose averaged 125 mg/dL. At that point, Frank started using the modified Tabata exercise approach two days a week, using a stationary exercise bike he had in his basement. He also added 1,000 mg daily of L-carnitine to reduce blood glucose levels further and for heart health. He admitted that following the antiglycation eating program was "a bit difficult, especially since I really love fried foods," but that his wife was "holding me to it. Poached fish, soups, and oatmeal are now a big part of my diet."

Nine months after he was first diagnosed with type 2 diabetes, Frank weighs in at 205 pounds, his Hb A_{1c} is 6.2 percent, and his fasting glucose level averages 115 mg/dL. His triglycerides have dropped to 150 mg/dL, and his total cholesterol hovers around 198 mg/dL. "I still have a way to go," he says, "but I definitely feel like I have a handle on it now."

Endnotes

INTRODUCTION

www.diabetes.org/diabetesnewsarticle.jsp?storyId=1535
1710&filename=20070623/ADA200706231182625856
41EDIT.xml
.

CHAPTER 1

Boyle JP et al. Projection of diabetes burden through 2050: Impact of changing demography and disease prevalence in the U.S. *Diabetes Care* 2001; 24(11):1936-40.

Clarke SD. Polyunsaturated fatty acid regulation of gene transcription: A mechanism to improve energy balance and insulin resistance. *Br J Nutr* 2000 Mar; 83 Suppl 1:S59-66.

Esposito K et al. Effect of a Mediterranean-style diet on endothelial dysfunction and markers of vascular inflammation in the metabolic syndrome: A randomized trial. *JAMA* 2004 Sept 22; 292(12):1440-46.

Forbes JM et al. Below the radar: Advanced glycation end products that detour "around the side." Is HbA1c not an accurate predictor of long term progression and glycaemic control in diabetes? *Clin Biochem Rev* 2006 Nov; 26(4):123-34.

Goldberg T et al. Advanced glycation end products in commonly consumed foods. *J Am Diet Assoc* 2004 Aug; 104(8):1287-91.

Gu K et al. Mortality in adults with and without diabetes in a national cohort of the U.S. population, 1971-1993. *Diabetes Care* 1998 Jul; 21(7):1138-45.

Inoguchi T et al. High glucose level and free fatty acid stimulate reactive oxygen species production through protein kinase C-dependent activation of NAD(P)H oxidase in cultured vascular cells. *Diabetes* 2000 Nov; 49(11):1939-45.

Kaufman FR. Type 2 diabetes mellitus in children and youth: A new epidemic. *J Pediatr Endocrinol Metab* 2002 May; 15 Suppl 2:737-44.

Laight DW et al. Endothelial dysfunction accompanies a pro-oxidant, pro-diabetic challenge in the insulin resistant, obese Zucker rat in vivo. *Eur J Pharmacol* 2000 Aug 18; 402(1-2):95-99.

Li SY et al. High-fat diet enhances visceral advanced glycation end products, nuclear O-Glc-Noc modification, p38 mitogen-activated protein kinase activation and apoptosis. *Diabetes Obes Metab* 2005 Jul; 7(4):448-54.

Mills, R. Will diabetes research lead to a cure for aging? www.delano.com/Articles/Aging-and-diabetes.html

Miyata T et al. Angiotensin II receptor blockers and angiotensin converting enzyme inhibitors: Implication of radical scavenging and transition metal chelation in inhibition of advanced glycation end product formation. *Arch Biochem Biophys* 2003 Nov 1; 419(1):50-54.

National Institutes of Diabetes and Digestive and Kidney Diseases: http://diabetes.niddk.nih.gov/dm/pubs/insulinresistance/

Ohara Y et al. Hypercholesterolemia increases endothelial superoxide anion production. *J Clin Invest* 1993 Jun; 91(6):2546-51.

Paolisso G, Giugliano D. Oxidative stress and insulin action: Is there a relationship? *Diabetologia* 1996; 39:357-63.

Reaven G. Insulin resistance, type 2 diabetes mellitus, and cardiovascular disease: The end of the beginning. *Circulation* 2005 Nov 15; 112(20):3030-2.

Shigenaga MK et al. Oxidative damage and mitochondrial decay in aging. *Proc Natl Acad Sci USA* 1994 Nov 8; 91(23):10771-8.

Sonoki K et al. Decreased lipid peroxidation following periodontal therapy in type 2 diabetic patients. *J Periodontology* 2006; 77 (11):1907-13.

Uribarri J et al. Dietary-derived advanced glycation end products are major contributors to the body's AGE pool and induce inflammation in healthy subjects. *Ann NY Acad Sci* 2005; 1043:461-66.

Vaughan N et al. A 5-year prospective study of diabetes and hearing loss in a veteran population. *Otol Neurotol* 2006 Jan; 27(1):37-43.

Vlassara H et al. Inflammatory mediators are induced by dietary glycotoxins, a major risk factor for diabetic angiopathy. *Proc Natl Acad Sci USA* 2002 Nov 26; 99(24):15596-601.

Wiernsperger NF. Oxidative stress as a therapeutic target in diabetes: Revisiting the controversy. *Diabetes Metab* 2003; 29:579-85.

Zhang J et al. Hostility and urine norepinephrine interact to predict insulin resistance: The VA Normative Aging Study. *Psychosom Med* 2006; 68:718-26.

CHAPTER 2

American Heart Association: www.americanheart.org/presenter. jhtml?identifier=3039230

Audebert Heinrich J. Predictors of progression in lacunar stroke. *Abstracts of the International Stroke Conference* 2000 32:347-c.

Bjornholt JV et al. Fasting blood glucose: An underestimated risk factor for cardiovascular death. Results from a 22-year follow-up of healthy nondiabetic men. *Diabetes Care* 1999 Jan; 22(1):45-49.

Boney CM et al. Metabolic syndrome in childhood: association with birth weight, maternal obesity and gestational diabetes mellitus. *Pediatrics* 2005 Mar; 115(3):e290-96.

Chen Jiunn-Rong. Dilatation of common carotid artery is strongly associated with cerebral ischemic stroke with or without the presence of carotid atherosclerosis. *Abstracts of the International Stroke Conference* 2000 32:365-d.

Chyi-Huey Bai et al. Relations between coagulation profiles, lipid profiles, and other risk factors with risk of first-ever ischemic stroke: A novel case-control study. *Abstracts of the International Stroke Conference* 2000 32:367-b Poster Presentation. P 156.

de Ferranti SD et al. Inflammation and changes in metabolic syndrome abnormalities in U.S. adolescents: Findings from the 1988-1994 and 1999-2000 National Health and Nutrition Examination Surveys. *Clin Chem* 2006; 52:1325-30.

Isomaa B et al. Cardiovascular morbidity and mortality associated with the metabolic syndrome. *Diabetes Care* 2001 Apr; 24(4):683-89.

Lakka HM et al. The metabolic syndrome and total and cardiovascular disease mortality in middle-aged men. *JAMA* 2002 Dec 4; 288(21):2709-16.

Malik S et al. Impact of the metabolic syndrome on mortality from coronary heart disease, cardiovascular disease, and all causes in United States adults. *Circulation* 2004 Sep 7; 110(10):1245-50.

Nakanishi N et al. Components of the metabolic syndrome as predictors of cardiovascular disease and type 2 diabetes in middle-aged Japanese men. *Diabetes Res Clin Pract* 2004 Apr; 64(1):59-70.

National Heart, Lung, and Blood Institute statistics: www.nhlbi.nih.gov/hbp/hbp/whathbp.htm

Reaven G. The metabolic syndrome: Is this diagnosis necessary? *Am J Clin Nutr* 2006 Jun; 83(6):1237-47.

Selvin E et al. Glycemic control and coronary heart disease risk in persons with and without diabetes: The atherosclerosis risk in communities study. *Arch Intern Med* 2005 Sep 12; 165(16):1910-6.

Tapsell LC et al. Including walnuts in a low-fat/modified-fat diet improves HDL cholesterol-to-total cholesterol ratios in patients with type 2 diabetes. *Diabetes Care* 2004; 27:2777-83.

Trouillas P. The "making" of a parenchymal hematoma. An early coagulopathy and specific risk factors contribute to grave intracerebral bleeding after intravenous rtPA thrombolysis. *Abstracts of the International Stroke Conference* 2000 32:345-a.

Wang Y et al. Comparison of abdominal adiposity and overall obesity in predicting risk of type 2 diabetes among men. *Am J Clin Nutr* 2005 Mar; 81(3):555-63.

Weiss R et al. Obesity and the metabolic syndrome in children and adolescents. *NEJM* 2004; 350:2362-74.

CHAPTER 3

American Association of Periodontology. Diabetes and periodontal diseases (position paper). *J Periodontol* 1999; 70:935-49.

American Diabetes Association. Management of dyslipidemia in adults with diabetes. *Diabetes Care* 2000; 23 Suppl 1:557-60.

Brownlee M. Glycation products and the pathogenesis of diabetic complications. *Diabetes Care* 1992; 15:1835-43.

Brownlee M. Glycation and diabetic complications. *Diabetes* 1994; 43:836-41.

de Boer IH et al. Central obesity, incident microalbuminuria, and change in creatinine clearance in the epidemiology of diabetes interventions and complications study. *J Am Soc Nephrol* 2006 Dec 6.

Dhindsa S et al. Frequent occurrence of hypogonadotropic hypogonadism in type 2 diabetes. *J Clin Endocrinol Metab* 2004 Nov; 89(11):5462-68.

Dugy JJ et al. Diabetic neuropathy: An intensive review. *Am J Health Syst Pharm* 2004 Jan 15; 61(2):160-73.

Galili D et al. Oral and dental complications associated with diabetes and their treatment. *Compendium* 1994; 15:496-509.

Gami AS et al. Metabolic syndrome and risk of incident cardiovascular events and death: A systematic review and meta-analysis of longitudinal studies. *J Am Coll Cardiol* 2007 Jan 30; 49(4):403-14.

Geiss LS et al. Elevated blood pressure among U.S. adults with diabetes, 1988-1994. *Am J Prev Med* 2002 Jan; 22(1):42-48.

Gotto AM. Triglycerides: The forgotten risk factor. *Circulation* 1998; 97(11):1027-28.

Hu FB et al. Elevated risk of cardiovascular disease prior to clinical diagnosis of type 2 diabetes. *Diabetes Care* 2002; 25:1129-34. At: www.medscape.com/viewarticle/439891

Jeerakathil T et al. Short-term risk for stroke is doubled in persons with newly treated type 2 diabetes compared with persons without diabetes. *Stroke* 2007 Jun; 38:1739-43.

Lau DCW et al. Adipokines: Molecular links between obesity and atherosclerosis. *Am J Physiol Heart Circ Physiol* 2005; 288: H2031-41.

Locatelli F et al. The importance of diabetic nephropathy in current nephrological practice. *Nephrol Dial Transplant* 2003 Sep; 18(9):1716-25.

Malkin CJ et al. Testosterone as a protective factor against atherosclerosis—immunomodulation and influence upon plaque development and stability. *J Endocrinol* 2003 Sep; 178(3):373-80.

Mangrum A, Bakris GL. Predictors of renal and cardiovascular mortality in patients with non-insulin-dependent diabetes: A brief overview of microalbuminuria and insulin resistance. *J Diabetes Complications* 1997 Nov-Dec; 11(6):352-57.

Muis MJ et al. High cumulative insulin exposure: A risk factor of atherosclerosis in type 1 diabetes? *Atherosclerosis.* 2005 Jul; 181(1):185-92.

Musicki B et al. Inactivation of phosphorylated endothelial nitric oxide synthase (Ser-1177) by O-GlcNAc in diabetes-associated erectile dysfunction. *Proc Natl Acad Sci USA* 2005 Aug 16; 102(33):11870-5.

Selvin E et al. Prevalence and risk factors for erectile dysfunction in the US. *Am J Med* 2007 Feb; 120(2):151-57.

Sharrett AR et al. Associations of lipoprotein cholesterols, apolipoproteins A-I and B, and triglycerides with carotid atherosclerosis and coronary heart disease. The Atherosclerosis Risk in Communities (ARIC) Study. *Arterioscler Thromb* 1994 Jul; 14(7):1098-104.

Stochmal E et al. Association of coronary atherosclerosis with insulin resistance in patients with impaired glucose tolerance. *Acta Cardiol* 2005 Jun; 60(3):325-31.

Uribarri J et al. Restriction of dietary glycotoxins reduces excessive age glycated end products in renal failure patients. *J Am Soc Nephrol* 2003; 14:728-31.

van Gaal LF et al. Mechanisms linking obesity with cardiovascular disease. *Nature* 2006 Dec 14; 444(7121):875-80.

Verma S. C-reactive protein incites atherosclerosis. *Can J Cardiol* 2004 Aug; 20 Suppl B29B-31B.

Xie LQ, Wang X. C-reactive protein and atherosclerosis. *Sheng Li Ke Xue Jin Zhan* 2004 Apr; 35(2):113-18.

Zheng H et al. Lack of central nitric oxide triggers erectile dysfunction in diabetes. *Am J Physiol Regul Integr Comp Physiol* 2007 Mar; 292(3):R1158-64.

CHAPTER 4

Diabetes Prevention Program Research Group. Reduction in the incidence of type 2 diabetes with lifestyle intervention or metformin. *N Engl J Med* 2002 Feb 7; 346(6):393-403.

Gotto AM Jr. Triglyceride as a risk factor for coronary artery disease. *Am J Cardiol* 1998 Nov 5; 82(9A):22Q-25Q.

Gotto AM Jr. Triglyceride: The forgotten risk factor. *Circulation* 1998; 97(11):1027-28.

Kapoor S et al. Testosterone replacement therapy improves insulin resistance, glycaemic control, visceral adiposity and hypercholesterolaemia in hypogonadal men with type 2 diabetes. *Eur J Endocrinol* 2006 Jun; 154(6):899-906.

Marin et al. The effects of testosterone treatment on body composition and metabolism in middle-aged obese men. *Int J Obes Relat Metab Disord* 1992 Dec; 16(12):991-97.

McLaughlin T et al. Use of metabolic markers to identify overweight individuals who are insulin resistant. *Ann Intern Med* 2003 Nov 18; 139(10):802-9.

Nissen SE et al. Statin therapy, LDL cholesterol, C-reactive protein, and coronary artery disease. *N Engl J Med* 2005 Jan 6; 352(1):29-38.

Ridker PM et al. C-reactive protein levels and outcomes after statin therapy. *N Engl J Med* 2005 Jan 6; 352(1):20-28.

CHAPTER 5

Alfenas RC, Mattes RD. Influence of glycemic index/load on glycemic response, appetite, and food intake in healthy humans. *Diabetes Care* 2005 Sep; 28(9):2123-39.

Bergner P. *The healing power of minerals, special nutrients and trace elements.* Rocklin CA: Prima Publishing, 1997, p. 312.

Connor SL, Connor WE. Are fish oils beneficial in the prevention and treatment of coronary artery disease? *Am J Clin Nutr* 1997 Oct; 66(4 Suppl):1020S-1031S.

Ello-Martin et al. Dietary energy density in the treatment of obesity: A year-long trial comparing 2 weight-loss diets. *Am J Clin Nutr* 2007 Jun; 85(6):1465-77.

Erkkila AT, Lichtenstein AH. Fiber and cardiovascular disease risk: How strong is the evidence? *J Cardiovasc Nurs* 2006 Jan-Feb; 21(1):3-8.

Fatty fish consumption and ischemic heart disease mortality in older adults: The cardiovascular heart study. Presented at the American Heart Association's 41st annual conference on cardiovascular disease epidemiology and prevention. *AHA* 2001.

Finot PA, Magnenat E. Metabolic transit of early and advanced Maillard products. *Prog Food Nutr Sci* 1981; 5(1-6):193-207.

Foster-Powell K et al. International table of glycemic index and glycemic load values: 2002. *Am J Clin Nutr* 76:5-56.

Goldberg T et al. Advanced glycation end products in commonly consumed foods. *J Am Diet Assoc* 2004 Aug; 104(8):1287-91.

Harper CR, Jacobson TA. The fats of life: The role of omega-3 fatty acids in the prevention of coronary heart disease. *Arch Intern Med* 2001; 161(18):2185-92.

Koschinsky T et al. Orally absorbed reactive glycation products (glycotoxins): An environmental risk factor in diabetic nephropathy. *Proc Natl Acad Sci USA* 1997 Jun 10; 94(12):6474-79.

Ledikwe et al. Reductions in dietary energy density are associated with weight loss in overweight and obese participants in the PRE-MIER trial. *Am J Clin Nutr* 2007 May; 85(5):1212-21.

Lovejoy et al. Effects of diets enriched in saturated (palmitic), monounsaturated (oleic), or trans (elaidic) fatty acids on insulin sensitivity and substrate oxidation in healthy adults. *Diabetes Care* 2002 Aug; 25(8):1283-88.

Mayer-Davis EJ et al. Towards understanding of glycaemic index and glycaemic load in habitual diet: Associations with measures of glycaemia in the Insulin Resistance Atherosclerosis Study. *Br J Nutr* 2006 Feb; 95(2):397-405.

O'Brien J, Morrissey PA. Nutritional and toxicological aspects of the Maillard browning reaction in foods. *Crit Rev Food Sci Nutr* 1989; 28(3):211-48.

Rimm EB et al. Vegetable, fruit, and cereal fiber intake and risk of coronary heart disease among men. *JAMA* 1996 Feb 14; 275(6):447-51.

Salas-Salvado J et al. Components of the Mediterranean-type food pattern and serum inflammatory markers among patients at high risk for cardiovascular disease. *Eur J Clin Nutr* 2007 Apr 18.

Stark AH, Madar Z. Olive oil as a functional food: Epidemiology and nutritional approaches. *Nutr Rev* 2002 Jun; 60(6):170-76.

Sugano M. Characteristics of fats in Japanese diets and current recommendations. *Lipids* 1996 Mar; 31 Suppl:S283-86.

Tapsell LC et al. Including walnuts in a low-fat/modified-fat diet improves HDL cholesterol-to-total cholesterol ratios in patients with type 2 diabetes. *Diabetes Care* 2004; 27:2777-83.

U.S. Senate, 1936, "Modern Muscle Men," *Proper Food Mineral Balances,* Charles Northen, 74th Cong, 2d sess. Serial set 10016.

Vlassara H et al. Inflammatory mediators are induced by dietary glycotoxins, a major risk factor for diabetic angiopathy. *Proc Natl Acad Sci USA* 2002 Nov 26; 99(24):15596-601.

Williams CM. Beneficial nutritional properties of olive oil: Implications for postprandial lipoproteins and factor VII. *Nutr Metab Cardiovasc Dis* 2001 Aug; 11 Suppl 4:51-56.

CHAPTER 6

Jiang R et al. Nut and peanut butter consumption and risk of type 2 diabetes in women. *JAMA* 2002 Nov 27; 288:2554-60.

Tapsell LC et al. Including walnuts in a low-fat/modified-fat diet improves HDL cholesterol-to-total cholesterol ratios in patients with type 2 diabetes. *Diabetes Care* 2004 Dec; 7(12):2777-83.

CHAPTER 7

Cauza E et al. The relative benefits of endurance and strength training on the metabolic factors and muscle function of people with type 2 diabetes mellitus. *Arch Phys Med Rehabil* 2005 Aug; 86(8):1527-33.

Cauza E et al. The metabolic effects of long term exercise in type 2 diabetes patients. *Wien Med Wochenschr* 2006 Sep; 156(17-18):515-19.

Eriksson J et al. Resistance training in the treatment of non-insulin dependent diabetes mellitus. *Intl J Sports Med* 1997; 18:242-46.

Faigenbaum AD et al. Acute effects of different warmup protocols on fitness performance in children. *J Strength Cond Res* 2005 May; 19(2):376-81.

Ishii T et al. Resistance training improves insulin sensitivity in NIDDM subjects without altering maximal oxygen uptake. *Diabetes Care* 1998; 21:1353-55.

Little T, Williams AG. Effects of differential stretching protocols during warmups on high-speed motor capacities in professional soccer players. *J Strength Cond Res* 2006 Feb; 20(1):203-7.

Melov S et al. Resistance exercise reverses aging in human skeletal muscle. 2007; PLoS ONE 2(5): e465. doi:10.1371/journal.pone.0000465

Puetz TW et al. Effects of chronic exercise on feelings of energy and fatigue: A quantitative synthesis. *Psychological Bulletin* 2006 Nov; 132(6):866-76.

Smith TC et al. Walking decreased risk of cardiovascular disease mortality in older adults with diabetes. *J Clin Epidemiol* 2007 Mar; 60(3):309-17.

Tabata I et al. Effects of moderate-intensity endurance and high-intensity intermittent training on anaerobic capacity and VO2max. *Med Sci Sports Exerc* 1996 Oct; 28(10):1327-30.

CHAPTER 8

Abidoff MT. Special clinical report on effects of glucose-6-phos-phatase on human subjects. Russian Ministry of Health, Moscow, 1999; unpublished study.

Alhamdani MS et al. Decreased formation of advanced glycation end-products in peritoneal fluid by carnosine and related peptides. *Perit Dial Int* 2007 Jan-Feb; 27(1):86-89.

American Diabetes Association. 66th Scientific Sessions, 2006, Abstract 327-OR.

Anderson RA. Chromium as an essential nutrient for humans. *Regul Toxicol Pharmacol* 1997 Aug; 26(1Pt 2):S35-41.

Anderson RA et al. Isolation and characterization of polyphenol type-A polymers from cinnamon with insulin-like biological activity. *J Agric Food Chem* 2004 Jan 14; 52(1):65-70.

Appel LJ. Nonpharmacologic therapies that reduce blood pressure: A fresh perspective. *Clin Cardiol* 1999; 22 Suppl. III:1-5.

Attele AS et al. Antidiabetic effects of *Panax ginseng* berry extract and the identification of an effective component. *Diabetes* 2002 Jun; 51(6):1851-58.

Aviram M, Dornfeld L. Pomegranate juice consumption inhibits serum angiotensin converting enzyme activity and reduces systolic blood pressure. *Atherosclerosis* 2001 Sep; 158(1):195-98.

Aviram M et al. Pomegranate juice consumption for 3 years by patients with carotid artery stenosis reduces common carotid intima-media thickness, blood pressure and LDL oxidation. *Clin Nutr* 2004 Jun; 23(3):423-33.

Babu PV et al. Therapeutic effect of green tea extract on oxidative stress in aorta and heart of streptozotocin diabetic rats. *Chem Biol Interact* 2006 Aug 25; 162(2):114-20.

Babu PV et al. Cinnamaldehyde—a potential antidiabetic agent. *Phytomedicine* 2007 Jan; 14(1):15-22.

Babu PV et al. Green tea attenuates diabetes induced Maillard-type fluorescence and collagen cross-linking in the heart of streptozotocin diabetic rats. *Pharmacol Res* 2007 May; 55(5):433-40.

Basu R et al. Obesity and type 2 diabetes impair insulin-induced suppression of glycogenolysis as well as gluconeogenesis. *Diabetes* 2005 Jul; 54(7):1942-48.

Belobrajdic DP et al. A high-whey-protein diet reduces body weight gain and alters insulin sensitivity relative to red meat in Wistar rats. *J Nutr* 2004 Jun; 134(6):1454-58.

Best L et al. Curcumin induces electrical activity in rat pancreatic beta-cells by activating the volume regulated anion channel. *Biochem Pharmacol* 2007; 73:1768-75.

Boudou P et al. Hyperglycaemia acutely decreases circulating dehydroepiandrosterone levels in healthy men. *Clin Endocrinol (Oxf)* 2006 Jan; 64(1):46-52.

Breithaupt-Grogler K et al. Dose-proportionality of oral thioctic acid—coincidence of assessments via pooled plasma and individual data. *Eur J Pharm Sci* 1999 Apr; 8(1):57-65.

Broadhurst CL, Domenico P. Clinical studies on chromium picolinate supplementation in diabetes mellitus—A review. *Diabetes Technol Ther* 2006 Dec; 8(6):677-87.

Brownson C, Hipkiss AR. Carnosine reacts with a glycated protein. *Free Radic Biol Med* 2000 May 15; 28(10):1564-70.

Cefalu WT, Hu FB. Role of chromium in human health and in diabetes. *Diabetes Care* 2004; 27:2741-51.

Ceylan-Isik AF et al. High-dose benfotiamine rescues cardiomyocyte contractile dysfunction in streptozotocin-induced diabetes mellitus. *J Appl Physiol* 2006 Jan; 100(1):150-56.

Cheng JT, Liu IM. Stimulatory effect of caffeic acid on alpha1A-adrenoceptors to increase glucose uptake into cultured C2C12 cells. *Naunyn Schmiedeberg's Arch Pharmacol* 2000 Aug; 362(2):122-27.

Cloarec M et al. GliSODin, a vegetal sod with gliadin, as preventative agent vs. atherosclerosis, as confirmed with carotid ultrasound-B imaging. *Allerg Immunol (Paris)* 2007 Feb; 39(2):45-50.

Connor SL, Connor WE. Are fish oils beneficial in the prevention and treatment of coronary artery disease? *Am J Clin Nutr* 1997; 66 Suppl:1020S-31S.

Covington MB. Omega-3 fatty acids. *Am Fam Physician* 2004; 70:133-40.

Crespy V, Williamson G. A review of the health effects of green tea catechins in vivo animal models. *J Nutr* 2004 Dec; 134 Suppl:3431S-40S.

Davini P et al. Controlled study on L-carnitine therapeutic efficacy in post-infarction. *Drugs Exp Clin Res* 1992; 18(8):355-65.

De Gaetano A et al. Carnitine increases glucose disposal in humans. *J Am Coll Nutr* 1999; 18:289-95.

Dewailly E. n-3 fatty acids and cardiovascular disease risk factors among the Inuit of Nunavik. *Am J Clin Nutr* 2001 Oct; 74(4):464-73.

Dewailly E. Fish consumption and blood lipids in three ethnic groups of Quebec (Canada). *Lipids* 2003 Apr; 38(4):359-65.

Dincer Y et al. Effect of oxidative stress on glutathione pathway in red blood cells from patients with insulin-dependent diabetes mellitus. *Metabolism* 2002 Oct; 51(10):1360-62.

Doggrell SA. Alpha-lipoic acid, an anti-obesity agent? *Expert Opin Investig Drugs* 2004 Dec; 13(12):1641-43.

Dulloo AG et al. Efficacy of a green tea extract rich in catechin polyphenols and caffeine in increasing 24-h energy expenditure and fat oxidation in humans. *Am J Clin Nutr* 1999; 70:1040-45.

Eibl NL et al. Hypomagnesemia in type II diabetes: Effect of a 3-month replacement therapy. *Diabetes Care* 1995 Feb; 18(2):188-92.

Esmaillzadeh A et al. Cholesterol-lowering effect of concentrated pomegranate juice consumption in type II diabetic patients with hyperlipidemia. *Int J Vitam Nutr Res* 2006 May; 76(3):147-51.

Frid AH et al. Effect of whey on blood glucose and insulin responses to composite breakfast and lunch meals in type 2 diabetic subjects. *Am J Clin Nutr* 2005 Jul; 82(1):69-75.

Friedberg CE et al. Fish oil and glycemic control in diabetes: A meta-analysis. *Diabetes Care* 1998; 21:494-500.

Gross CJ et al. Uptake of L-carnitine, D-carnitine and acetyl-L-carnitine by isolated guinea-pig enterocytes. *Biochim Biophys Acta* 1986; 886(3):425-33.

Hagen TM et al. Feeding acetyl-L-carnitine and lipoic acid to old rats significantly improves metabolic function while decreasing oxidative stress. *Proc Natl Acad Sci USA* 2002; 99(4):1870-75.

Halat KM, Dennehy CE. Botanicals and dietary supplements in diabetic peripheral neuropathy. *J Am Board Fam Pract* 2003 Jan-Feb; 16(1):47-57.

Hall WL et al. Casein and whey exert different effects on plasma amino acid profiles, gastrointestinal hormone secretion and appetite. *Br Nutr* 2003 Feb; 89(2):239-48.

Hama T et al. Intestinal absorption of beta-alanine, anserine and carnosine in rats. *J Nutr Sci Vitaminol* (Tokyo) 1976; 22(2):147-57.

Harper CR, Jacobson TA. The fats of life: The role of omega-3 fatty acids in the prevention of coronary heart disease. *Arch Intern Med* 2001; 161(18):2185-92.

Harris WS. Extending the cardiovascular benefits of omega-3 fatty acids. *Curr Atheroscler Rep* 2005 Sep; 7(5):375-80.

Haupt E et al. Benfotiamine in the treatment of diabetic polyneuropathy—a three-week randomized, controlled pilot study (BEDIP study). *Int J Clin Pharmacol Ther* 2005 Feb; 43(2):71-77.

He K et al. Magnesium intake and incidence of metabolic syndrome among young adults. *Circulation* Apr 2006; 113:1675-82.

Hemmerle H et al. Chlorogenic acid and synthetic chlorogenic acid derivatives: Novel inhibitors of hepatic glucose-6-phosphate translocase. *J Med Chem* 1997 Jan 17; 40(2):137-45.

Hendler SS, Rorvik DR, eds. *PDR for Nutritional Supplements.* Montvale: Medical Economics Co., Inc., 2001.

Hendry J. Chromium supplement controversy continues. *DOC News* 2006 June 1; 3(6):9.

Hipkiss AR. Carnosine, a protective, anti-aging peptide? *Int J Biochem Cell Biol* 1998 Aug; 30(8):863-68.

Hoskins JA. The occurrence, metabolism and toxicity of cinnamic acid and related compounds. *J Appl Toxicol* 1984 Dec; 4(6):283-92.

Hosoe K et al. Study on safety and bioavailability of ubiquinol (Kaneka QH) after single and 4-week multiple oral administration to healthy volunteers. *Regul Toxicol Pharmacol* 2006 Aug 17.

Hu FB et al. Dietary intake of alpha-linolenic acid and risk of fatal ischemic heart disease among women. *Am J Clin Nutr* 1999; 69:890-97.

Hypponen E et al. Intake of vitamin D and risk of type 1 diabetes: A birth-cohort study. *Lancet* 2001 Nov 3; 358(9292):1500-3.

Imparl-Radosevich J et al. Regulation of PTP-1 and insulin receptor kinase by fractions from cinnamon: Implications for cinnamon regulation of insulin signaling. *Horm Res* 1998 Sep; 50(3):177-82.

Institute of Medicine. *Dietary Reference Intakes for vitamin A, vitamin K, arsenic, boron, chromium, copper, iodine, iron, manganese, molybdenum, nickel, silicon, vanadium, and zinc.* Washington, DC: National Academy Press, 2001.

Janssen B et al. Carnosine as a protective factor in diabetic nephropathy: Association with a leucine repeat of the carnosinase gene CNDP1. *Diabetes* 2005 Aug; 54(8):2320-7.

Johnston KL et al. Coffee acutely modifies gastrointestinal hormone secretion and glucose tolerance in humans: Glycemic effects of chlorogenic acid and caffeine. *Am J Clin Nutr* 2003 Oct; 78(4):728-33.

Kaneka Corp. Plasma levels of CoQ10 for ubiquinol increased dose dependently. Unpublished data.

Kaneka Corp. Ubiquinol has a higher bioavailability compared to ubiquinone. Unpublished data.

Kapoor D et al. Androgens, insulin resistance and vascular disease in men. *Clin Endocrinol (Oxf)* 2005 Sep; 63(3):239-50.

Khan A et al. Cinnamon improves glucose and lipids of people with type 2 diabetes. *Diabetes Care* 2003 Dec; 26(12):3215-18.

Kim MJ et al. Inhibitory effects of epicatechin on interleukin-1-beta-induced inducible nitric oxide synthase expression in RINm5F cells and rat pancreatic islets by down-regulation of NF-kappaB activation. *Biochem Pharmacol* 2004 Nov 1; 68(9):1775-85.

Kono S et al. Green tea consumption and serum lipid profiles: A cross-sectional study in northern Kyushu, Japan. *Prev Med* 1992 Jul; 21(4):526-31.

Kowluru RA, Kanwar M. Effects of curcumin on retinal oxidative stress and inflammation in diabetes. *Nutr Metab (Lond)* 2007 Apr 16; 4:8.

Kris-Etherton P et al. AHA Science Advisory: Lyon Diet Heart Study. Benefits of a Mediterranean-style, National Cholesterol Education Program/American Heart Association Step I dietary pattern on cardiovascular disease. *Circulation* 2001; 103:1823.

Kumar PA et al. Modulation of alpha-crystallin chaperone activity in diabetic rat lens by curcumin. *Mol Vis* 2005 Jul 26; 11:561-68.

Langsjoen PH, Langsjoen AM. Overview of the use of CoQ10 in cardiovascular disease. *Biofactor* 1999; 9(2-4):273-84.

Lapenna D et al. Dihydro-lipoic acid inhibits 15-lipoxygenase-dependent lipid peroxidation. *Free Radic Biol Med* 2003 Dec 15; 35(10):1203-9.

Lee KW, Lip GY. The role of omega-3 fatty acids in the secondary prevention of cardiovascular disease. *QJM* 2003 Jul; 96(7):465-80.

Liu J et al. Memory loss in old rats is associated with brain mitochondrial decay and RNA/DNA oxidation: Partial reversal by feeding acetyl-L-carnitine and/or R-alpha-lipoic acid. *Proc Natl Acad Sci USA* 2002; 99(4):2356-61.

Lopez-Ridaura R et al. Magnesium intake and risk of type 2 diabetes in men and women. *Diabetes Care* 2004 Jan; 27(1):134-40.

Lum H, Roebuck KA. Oxidant stress and endothelial cell dysfunction. *Am J Physiol Cell Physiol* 2001 Apr; 280(4):C719-41.

Luo JZ, Luo L. American ginseng stimulates insulin production and prevents apoptosis through regulation of uncoupling protein-2 in cultured beta cells. *Evid Based Complement Alternat Med* 2006 Sep; 3(3):365-72.

Mahaba HM et al. Magnesium deficiency and other risk factors for diabetic retinopathy. *J Egypt Public Health Assoc* 2000; 75(3-4):323-33.

Mahesh T et al. Effect of photo-irradiated curcumin treatment against oxidative stress in streptozotocin-induced diabetic rats. *J Medic Food* 2005 Jun; 8(2):251-55.

Marin P et al. The effects of testosterone treatment on body composition and metabolism in middle-aged obese men. *Int J Obes Relat Metab Disord* 1992 Dec; 16(12):991-97.

Martin J et al. Chromium picolinate supplementation attenuates body weight gain and increases insulin sensitivity in subjects with type 2 diabetes. *Diabetes Care* 2006 Aug; 29(8):1826-32.

McKenney J, Sica D. Prescription omega-3 fatty acids for the treatment of hypertriglyceridemia. *Am J Health-System Pharm* 2007; 646:595-605.

Medina MC et al. Dehydroepiandrosterone increases beta-cell mass and improves the glucose-induced insulin secretion by pancreatic islets from aged rats. *FEBS Lett* 2006 Jan 9; 580(1):285-90.

Melhem MF et al. Alpha-lipoic acid attenuates hyperglycemia and prevents glomerular mesangial matrix expansion in diabetes. *J Am Soc Nephrol* 2002 Jan; 13(1):108-16.

Merck Manual online: www.merck.com/mmhe/sec02/ch019/ch019l.html

Mingrone G. Carnitine in type 2 diabetes. *Ann NY Acad Sci* 2004; 1033:99-107.

Mingrone G et al. L-carnitine improves glucose disposal in type 2 diabetic patients. *J Am Coll Nutr* 1999; 77-82.

Mita T et al. Eicosapentaenoic acid reduces the progression of carotid intima-media thickness in patients with type 2 diabetes. *Atherosclerosis* 2007 Mar; 191(1):162-67.

Miura Y et al. Tea catechins prevent the development of atherosclerosis in apoprotein E-deficient mice. *J Nutr* 2001; 131(1):27-32.

Montori V et al. Fish oil supplementation in type 2 diabetes: A quantitative systematic review. *Diabetes Care* 2000; 23:1407-15.

Mori TA. Omega-3 fatty acids and hypertension in humans. *Clin Exp Pharmacol Physiol* 2006 Sep; 33(9):842-46.

Mori TA et al. Dietary fish as a major component of a weight-loss diet: Effect on serum lipids, glucose, and insulin metabolism in overweight hypertensive subjects. *Am J Clin Nutr* 1999; 70:817-25.

Morris MC, Sacks F, Rosner B. Does fish oil lower blood pressure? A meta-analysis of controlled trials. *Circulation* 1993; 88:523-33.

Munch G et al. Influence of advanced glycation end-products and AGE-inhibitors on nucleation-dependent polymerization of beta-amyloid peptide. *Biochim Biophys Acta* 1997 Feb 27; 1360(1):17-29.

Murase T et al. Beneficial effects of tea catechins on diet-induced obesity: Stimulation of lipid catabolism in the liver. *Int J Obes Relat Metab Disord* 2002 Nov; 26(11):1459-64.

Negrisanu G et al. Effects of 3-month treatment with the antioxidant alpha-lipoic acid in diabetic peripheral neuropathy. *Rom J Intern Med* 1999 Jul-Sep; 37(3):297-306.

No authors listed. Benfotiamine—monograph. *Altern Med Rev* 2006 Sept; 11(3):238-42.

Paynter NP et al. Coffee and sweetened beverage consumption and the risk of type 2 diabetes mellitus: The atherosclerosis risk in communities study. *Am J Epidemiol* 2006 Dec 1; 164(11):1075-84.

Pereira M et al. Coffee consumption and risk of type 2 diabetes mellitus: An 11-year prospective study of 28,812 postmenopausal women. *Arch Intern Med* 2006; 166:1311-16.

Pi-Sunyer FX. The role of viscous soluble fiber in the metabolic control of diabetes. A review with special emphasis on cereals rich in beta-glucan. *Diabetes Care* 1997 Nov; 29(11):1774-80.

Pittas AG, Dawson-Hughes B et al. Vitamin D and calcium intake in relation to type 2 diabetes in women. *Diabetes Care* 2006 Mar; 29(3):650-56.

Pittas AG et al. The role of vitamin D and calcium in type 2 diabetes: A systematic review and meta-analysis. *J Clin Endocrinol Metab* 2007 Mar 27.

Queenan KM et al. Concentrated oat beta-glucan, a fermentable fiber, lowers serum cholesterol in hypercholesterolemic adults in a randomized controlled trial. *Nutr J* 2007 Mar 26; 6:6.

Rajasekar P, Anuradha CV. L-carnitine inhibits protein glycation in vitro and in vivo: Evidence for a role in diabetic management. *Acta Diabetol* 2007 Jul; 44(2):83-90.

Rashid I et al. Carnosine and its constituents inhibit glycation of low-density lipoproteins that promotes foam cell formation in vitro. *FEBS Lett* 2007 Mar 6; 581(5):1067-70.

Rizos I. Three-year survival of patients with heart failure caused by dilated cardiomyopathy and L-carnitine administration. *Am Heart J* 2000; 139(2 Pt 3):S120-23.

Rodriguez-Moran M and Guerrero-Romero F. Oral magnesium supplementation improves insulin sensitivity and metabolic control in type 2 diabetic subjects: A randomized double-blind controlled trial. *Diabetes Care* 2003 Apr; 26(4):1147-52.

Rosenblat M et al. Anti-oxidative effects of pomegranate juice (PJ) consumption by diabetic patients on serum and on macrophages. *Atherosclerosis* 2006 Aug; 187(2):363-71.

Sanchez-Ramirez GM et al. Benfotiamine relieves inflammatory and neuropathic pain in rats. *Eur J Pharmacol* 2006 Jan 13; 530(1-2):48-53.

SanGiovanni JD, Chew EY. The role of omega-3 long-chain polyunsaturated fatty acids in health and disease of the retina. *Prog Retin Eye Res* 2005 Jan; 24(1):87-138.

Savitha S, Panneerselvam C. Mitochondrial membrane damage during aging process in rat heart: Potential efficacy of L-carnitine and DL alpha lipoic acid. *Mech Ageing Dev* 2006; 127(4):349-55.

Schulze MB et al. Fiber and magnesium intake and incidence of type 2 diabetes: A prospective study and meta-analysis. *Arch Intern Med* 2007 May 14; 167(9):956-65.

Sethumadhavan S, Chinnakannu P. Carnitine and lipoic acid alleviates protein oxidation in heart mitochondria during aging process. *Biogerontology* 2006; 7(2):101-9.

Shults CW et al. Effects of coenzyme Q10 in early Parkinson disease: Evidence of slowing of the functional decline. *Arch Neurol* 2002 Oct; 59(10):1541-50.

Shults CW et al. Pilot trial of high dosages of coenzyme Q10 in patients with Parkinson's disease. *Exp Neurol* 2004 Aug; 188(2):491-94.

Sima AF et al. Acetyl-L-carnitine improves pain, nerve regeneration, and vibratory perception in patients with chronic diabetic neuropathy: An analysis of two randomized placebo-controlled trials. *Diabetes Care* 2005 Jan; 28(1):89-94.

Singer GM, Geohas J. The effect of chromium picolinate and biotin supplementation on glycemic control in poorly controlled patients with type 2 diabetes mellitus: A placebo-controlled, double-blinded, randomized trial. *Diabetes Technol Ther* 2006 Dec; 8(6):636-43.

Smith B et al. Does coffee consumption reduce the risk of type 2 diabetes in individuals with impaired glucose? *Diabetes Care* 2005; 29:2385-90.

Song DU et al. Effect of drinking green tea on age-associated accumulation of Maillard-type fluorescence and carbonyl groups in rat aortic and skin collagen. *Arch Biochem Biophys* 2002 Jan 15; 397(2):424-29.

Song EK et al. Epigallocatechin gallate prevents autoimmune diabetes induced by multiple low doses of streptozotocin in mice. *Arch Pharm Res* 2003 Jul; 26(7):559-63.

Song KH et al. Alpha-lipoic acid prevents diabetes mellitus in diabetes-prone obese rats. *Biochem Biophys Res Commun* 2005 Jan 7; 326(1):197-202.

Song Y et al. Dietary magnesium intake in relation to plasma insulin levels and risk of type 2 diabetes in women. *Diabetes Care* 2004 Jan; 27(1):59-65.

Stirban A et al. Benfotiamine prevents macro- and microvascular endothelial dysfunction and oxidative stress following a meal rich in advanced glycation end products in individuals with type 2 diabetes. *Diabetes Care* 2006; 29:2064-71.

Tosiello L. Hypomagnesemia and diabetes mellitus: A review of clinical implications. *Arch Intern Med* 1996 Jun 10; 156(11): 1143-48.

Uribarri et al. Circulating glycotoxins and dietary advanced glycation endproducts: Two links to inflammatory response, oxidative stress, and aging. *J Gerontol A Biol Sci Med Sci* 2007 Apr; 62(4):427-33.

Van Dam et al. Coffee, caffeine, and risk of type 2 diabetes: A prospective cohort study in younger and middle-aged US women. *Diabetes Care* 2006; 29:398-403.

Vlassara et al. *Proc Natl Acad Sci USA* 2002 Nov 26; 99(24):15596-601.

von Schacky C et al. The effect of dietary omega-3 fatty acids on coronary atherosclerosis: A randomized, double-blind, placebo-controlled trial. *Ann Intern Med* 1999; 130:554-62.

Vuksan V et al. Korean red ginseng (*Panax ginseng*) improves glucose and insulin regulation in well-controlled, type 2 diabetes: Results of a randomized, double-blind, placebo-controlled study of efficacy and safety. *Nutr Metab Cardiovasc Dis* 2006 Jul 21.

Weber C et al. Effect of dietary coenzyme Q10 as an antioxidant in human plasma. *Mol Aspects Med* 1994; 15 Suppls:97-102.

Wright E Jr. et al. Oxidative stress in type 2 diabetes: The role of fasting and postprandial glycaemia. *Int J Clin Pract* 2006 Mar; 60(3):308-14.

Wu S, Ren J. Benfotiamine alleviates diabetes-induced cerebral oxidative damage independent of advanced glycation endproduct, tissue factor and TNF-alpha. *Neurosci Lett* 2006 Feb 13; 394(2):158-62.

Xie JT et al. Antihyperglycemic effects of total ginsenosides from leaves and stem of *Panax ginseng*. *Acta Pharmacol Sin* 2005 Sep; 26(9):1104-10.

Yamashita R et al. Effects of dehydroepiandrosterone on gluconeogenic enzymes and glucose uptake in human hepatoma cell line, HepG2. *Endocr J* 2005 Dec; 52(6):727-33.

Yan J et al. Reduced coenzyme Q10 supplementation decelerates senescence in SAMP1 mice. *Exp Gerontol* 2006 Feb; 41(2):130-40.

Yang TT, Koo MW. Hypocholesterolemic effects of Chinese tea. *Pharmacol Res* 1997; 35(6):505-12.

Yang TTC, Koo MW. Chinese green tea lowers cholesterol level through an increase in fecal lipid excretion. *Life Sciences* 1999; 66(5):411-23.

Yokoyama M et al. Effects of eicosapentaenoic acid on major coronary events in hypercholesterolemic patients (JELIS): A randomized open-label, blinded endpoint analysis. *Lancet* 2007 Mar 31; 369(9567):1090-98.

Yu YM et al. Effects of young barley leaf extract and antioxidative vitamins on LDL oxidation and free radical scavenging activities in type 2 diabetes. *Diabetes Metab* 2002; 28:1262.

Yu YM et al. Effect of young barley leaf extract and adlay on plasma lipids and LDL oxidation in hyperlipidemic smokers. *Biol Pharm Bull* 2004; 27:802-5.

Ziegler D et al. Oral treatment with alpha lipoic acid improves symptomatic diabetic polyneuropathy: The SYDNEY 2 trial. *Diabetes Care* 2006 Nov; 29(11):2365-70.

CHAPTER 9

Clouse RE, Lustman PJ. Depression and coronary heart disease in women with diabetes. *Psychosom Med* 2003 May-Jun; 65(3):376-83.

DeRubeis RJ et al. Cognitive therapy vs medications in the treatment of moderate to severe depression. *Arch Gen Psychiatry* 2005 Apr; 62(4):409-16.

Eren I et al. The effect of depression on quality of life of patients with type II diabetes mellitus. *Depress Anxiety* 2007 Feb 20.

Feldman G. Cognitive and behavioral therapies for depression: Overview, new directions, and practical recommendations for dissemination. *Psychiatr Clin North Am* 2007 Mar; 30(1):39-50.

Georgiades A et al. Study presented at the American Psychosomatic Society annual meeting, Budapest, Hungary, March 2007.

Granath J et al. Stress management: A randomized study of cognitive behavioural therapy and yoga. *Cogn Behav Ther* 2006; 35(1):3-10.

Hollon SD et al. Prevention of relapse following cognitive therapy vs medications in moderate to severe depression. *Arch Gen Psychiatry* 2005 Apr; 62(4):417-22.

Innes KE et al. Risk indices associated with the insulin resistance syndrome, cardiovascular disease, and possible protection with yoga: A systematic review. *J Am Board Fam Pract* 2005 Nov-Dec; 18(6):491-519.

Knowler WC et al. Reduction in the incidence of type 2 diabetes with lifestyle intervention or metformin. *N Engl J Med* 2002 Feb 7; 346(6):393-403.

Ludman E et al. Panic episodes among patients with diabetes. *General Hospital Psychiatry* 2006; 28:475-81.

Lustman PJ, Clouse RE. Depression in diabetic patients: The relationship between mood and glycemic control. *J Diabetes Complications* 2005 Mar-Apr; 19(2):113-22.

Lustman PJ et al. Fluoxetine for depression in diabetes: A randomized double-blind placebo-controlled trial. *Diabetes Care* 2000 May; 23(5):618-23.

Lustman PJ, Clouse RE. Treatment of depression in diabetes: Impact on mood and medical outcome. *J Psychosom Res* 2002 Oct; 53(4):917-24.

Lustman PJ et al. Cognitive behavioral therapy for depression in type 2 diabetes mellitus: A randomized, controlled trial. *Ann Intern Med* 1998 Oct 15; 129(8):613-21.

Lustman PJ et al. Factors influencing glycemic control in type 2 diabetes during acute- and maintenance-phase treatment of major depressive disorder with bupropion. *Diabetes Care* 2007 Mar; 30(3):459-66.

Malhotra V et al. Effect of yoga asanas on nerve conduction in type 2 diabetes. *Indian J Physiol Pharmacol* 2002 Jul; 46(3):298-306.

McKellar JD et al. Depression increases diabetic symptoms by complicating patients' self-care adherence. *Diabetes Educ* 2004 May-Jun; 30(3):485-92.

Sephton SE et al. Mindfulness meditation alleviates depressive symptoms in women with fibromyalgia: Results of a randomized clinical trial. *Arthritis Rheum* 2007 Feb 15; 57(1):77-85.

Singh S et al. Role of yoga in modifying certain cardiovascular functions in type 2 diabetic patients. *J Assoc Physicians India* 2004 Mar; 52:203-6.

Smith A et al. Mindfulness-based cognitive therapy for recurring depression in older people: A qualitative study. *Aging Ment Health* 2007 May; 11(3):346-57.

Streeter CC et al. Yoga asana sessions increase brain GABA levels: A pilot study. *J Altern Complement Med* 2007 May; 13(4):419-26.

Surwit Richard S. *The Mind Body Diabetes Revolution.* New York: Free Press, 2004, p. 32.

Surwit RS, Feinglos MN. The effects of relaxations on glucose tolerance in non-insulin-dependent diabetes. *Diabetes Care* 1983 Mar-Apr; 6(2):176-79.

Surwit RS et al. Stress management improves long-term glycemic control in type 2 diabetes. *Diabetes Care* 2002 Jan; 25 (1):30-34.

CHAPTER 10

ALLHAT Officers et al. Major outcomes in high-risk hypertensive patients randomized to angiotensin-converting enzyme inhibitor or calcium channel blocker vs diuretic: The Antihypertensive and Lipid-Lowering Treatment to Prevent Heart Attack Trial (ALLHAT). *JAMA* 2002 Dec 18; 288(23):2981-97.

Aspirin inhibits the formation of pentosidine, a cross-linking advanced glycation end product, in collagen. *Diabetes Res Clin Pract* 2007 Aug; 77(2):337-40.

Cabrera-Rode et al. Effect of standard nicotinamide in the prevention of type 1 diabetes in first-degree relatives of persons with type 1 diabetes. *Autoimmunity* 2006 Jun; 39(4):333-40.

Cauley JA et al. Effects of estrogen plus progestin on risk of fracture and bone mineral density: The Women's Health Initiative randomized trial. *JAMA* 2003 Oct 1; 290(13):1729-38.

Colhoun HM et al. On behalf of the CARDS investigators. Primary prevention of cardiovascular disease with atorvastatin in type 2 diabetes in the Collaborative Atorvastatin Diabetes Study (CARDS): Multicentre randomised placebo-controlled trial. *Lancet* 2004; 364:685-96.

Corbett J et al. Aminoguanidine, a novel inhibitor of nitric oxide formation, prevents diabetic vascular dysfunction. *Diabetes* 1992; 41:552-56.

Dhindsa S et al. Frequent occurrence of hypogonadotropic hypogonadism in type 2 diabetes. *J Clin Endocrin Metab* 2004 Nov; 89(11):5462-68.

DPP-4 inhibitors Galvus and Januvia will be the first oral drugs tackling type 2 diabetes via the incretin response: How do they compare? On Hospitalpharma Web site: www.hospitalpharma.com/features/feature.asp?ROW_ID=908 27 Sept. 2006

Einhorn PT et al. The Antihypertensive and Lipid Lowering

Treatment to Prevent Heart Attack Trial (ALLHAT) Heart Failure Validation Study: Diagnosis and prognosis. *Am Heart J* 2007 Jan; 153(1):42-53.

Elliott WJ, Meyer PM. Incident diabetes in clinical trials of antihypertensive drugs: A network meta-analysis. *Lancet* 2007 Jan 20; 369(9557):201-7.

Forbes JM et al. Reduction of the accumulation of advanced glycation end products by ACE inhibition in experimental diabetic nephropathy. *Diabetes* 2002 Nov; 51(11):3274-82.

GlaxoSmithKline letter, Feb. 2007 at www.fda.gov/medwatch/safety/2007/Avandia_GSK_Ltr.pdf

Hammes HP et al. Aminoguanidine inhibits the development of accelerated diabetic retinopathy in the spontaneous hypertensive rat. *Diabetologia* 1994; 37:32-35.

Hedderson MM et al. Androgenicity of progestins in hormonal contraceptives and the risk of gestational diabetes mellitus. *Diabetes Care* 2007 May; 30(5):1062-68.

Isley WL. Hepatotoxicity of thiazolidinediones. *Expert Opin Drug Saf* 2003 Nov; 2(6):581-86.

Joshi SR. Metformin: Old wine in new bottle—evolving technology and therapy in diabetes. *J Assoc Physicians India* 2005 Nov; 53:963-72.

Kahn SE et al. Glycemic durability of rosiglitazone, metformin, or glyburide monotherapy. *N Engl J Med* 2006 Dec 7; 355(23):2427-43.

Kapoor D et al. Testosterone replacement therapy improves insulin resistance, glycaemic control, visceral adiposity and hypercholesterolaemia in hypogonadal men with type 2 diabetes. *Eur J Endocrinol* 2006 Jun; 154(6):899-906.

Kilhovd BK et al. Angiotensin-converting enzyme inhibition influences serum levels of advanced glycation end products in patients with coronary artery disease: Results from a HOPE substudy. *Heart Drug* 2003; 3:67-72.

Koro CE et al. Glycemic control from 1988 to 2000 among U.S.

adults diagnosed with type 2 diabetes: A preliminary report. *Diabetes Care* 2004; 27:17-20.

Malik S, Lopez V et al. Undertreatment of cardiovascular risk factors among persons with diabetes in the United States. *Diabetes Res Clin Pract* 2006 Nov 20.

Marcy TR et al. Second-generation thiazolidinediones and hepotototoxicity. *Ann Pharmacother* 2004 Sep; 38(9):1419-23.

Mayfield JA, White RD. Insulin therapy for type 2 diabetes: Rescue, augmentation and replacement of beta-cell function. *Am Fam Physician* 2004; 70:E489-500.

Miyata T et al. Angiotensin II receptor antagonists and angiotensin-converting enzyme inhibitors lower in vitro the formation of advanced glycation end products: Biochemical mechanisms. *J Am Soc Nephrol* 2002; 13:2478-87.

Nangaku M et al. Anti-hypertensive agents inhibit in vivo the formation of advanced glycation end products and improve renal damage in a type 2 diabetic nephropathy rat model. *J Am Soc Nephrol* 2003; 14:1212-22.

Nissen SE, Wolski K. Effect of rosiglitazone on the risk of myocardial infarction and death from cardiovascular causes. *N Engl J Med* 2007 May 21.

No authors listed. Effects of ramipril on cardiovascular and microvascular outcomes in people with diabetes mellitus: Results of the HOPE study and MICRO-HOPE substudy. Heart Outcomes Prevention Evaluation Study Investigators. *Lancet* 2000 Jan 22; 355 (9200):253-59.

Ryan AS et al. Hormone replacement therapy, insulin sensitivity, and abdominal obesity in postmenopausal women. *Diabetes Care* 2002 Jan; 25(1):127-33.

Soulis-Liparota T et al. Retardation by aminoguanidine of development of albuminuria, mesangial expansion and tissue fluorescence in streptozotocin induced diabetic rat. *Diabetes* 1991; 40:1328-34.

Tilton R et al. Prevention of diabetic vascular dysfunction by guanidines. Inhibition of nitric oxide synthase versus advanced glycation end-product formation. *Diabetes* 1993; 42:221-32.

Tsunekawa S et al. Protection of pancreatic beta-cells by exendin-4 may involve the reduction of endoplasmic reticulum stress; in vivo and in vitro studies. *J Endocrinol* 2007 Apr; 193(1):65-74.

Wajchenberg BL. Beta-cell failure in diabetes and preservation by clinical treatment. *Endocr Rev* 2007 Apr; 28(2):187-218.

Zhang XH et al. Testosterone restores diabetes-induced erectile dysfunction and sildenafil responsiveness in two distinct animal models of chemical diabetes. *J Sex Med* 2006 Mar; 3(2):253-64.

Glossary

ACE inhibitor: See angiotensin-converting enzyme.

advanced glycation end products (AGEs): Substances that form as the result of glycation and can cause significant damage to the body's cells and organs.

angiotensin-converting enzyme (ACE) inhibitor: A drug that inhibits ACE, which in turn helps reduce blood pressure by relaxing the arteries. ACE inhibitors are also used to treat congestive heart failure.

atherosclerosis: A disease in which fat accumulates in the medium- and large-sized arteries and impedes blood flow. It is a frequent complication of diabetes.

autonomic neuropathy: A disease of the nerves that usually affects the internal organs, including the cardiovascular system, the digestive tract, and the bladder. The affected nerves function automatically and so are not under voluntary control.

beta cell: A type of cell produced in the pancreas that produces and releases insulin, a hormone that controls the level of glucose in the blood.

blood glucose: The main sugar manufactured by the body from carbohydrates, fats, and proteins. It is the main source of energy for the body and is transported to all cells via the bloodstream.

blood glucose monitoring: A way to identify how much glucose is present in your blood. The most common way to perform home blood glucose monitoring is through the use of a test strip onto which you place a tiny drop of blood, usually taken from a fingertip. The strip is inserted into a meter, which reads the blood and shows the glucose level in a digital display.

calcium-channel blocker: A type of drug used to lower blood pressure.

cholesterol: A fatty substance manufactured by the liver and found in the blood, muscle, brain, and other tissues. Cholesterol can be both beneficial and damaging, depending on its level in the body and where it accumulates. High cholesterol is a risk factor for metabolic syndrome and heart disease.

congestive heart failure: Heart failure caused by an inability of the heart to pump, which results in fluid accumulating in the body. It typically develops gradually over several years, but it can also occur suddenly.

coronary disease: Condition caused by insufficient blood flow, which is the result of blocked and/or hardening blood vessels. People with diabetes are at high risk of developing coronary disease.

C-reactive protein: A substance created by the body in the presence of inflammation; thus elevated levels of C-reactive protein indicate increased inflammation in the body. Measuring C-reactive protein levels helps predict cardiovascular risk.

creatinine: A waste product of muscle metabolism. Measuring levels of creatinine is helpful in identifying and monitoring kidney function. Rising levels of creatinine indicate kidney disease or failure.

diabetic retinopathy: A disease that affects the small blood vessels of the retina of the eye. Blurred vision is one of the first symptoms of this disease. Progression of diabetic retinopathy can lead to more severely impaired vision or blindness.

diuretic: A drug or natural substance that increases the flow and elimination of urine.

fasting blood glucose test: A test that identifies how much glucose is in the bloodstream that is used to screen for prediabetes and diabetes. A blood sample is drawn after at least an eight-hour fast, and the results indicate the following: 99 mg/dL or less indicates no impaired fasting glucose; 100 to 126 mg/dL indicates prediabetes (impaired fasting glucose and a higher risk of developing diabetes); and greater than 126 mg/dL indicates diabetes.

fiber: A type of carbohydrate found in plant foods. There are two types of fiber: soluble, which dissolves in water and can help reduce blood fat and glucose levels; and insoluble, which assists the body in eliminating waste products.

fructose: A type of sugar found in fruit, vegetables, and honey. Fructose is available in a crystalline form (nearly 100 percent fructose) and as high-fructose (corn) syrup (approximately equal amounts of glucose and fructose).

galactose: A type of sugar manufactured by the body but also found in milk products and sugar beets.

gangrene: A condition in which the tissues die, usually caused by a loss of blood flow to the affected area of the body or by failing to recognize or treat an infection due to a lack of sensation in the affected area. Neuropathy in the lower leg, for example, can cause individuals to not feel a cut or wound in the foot that can then become infected and gangrenous, requiring amputation.

gene: A basic unit of heredity. Genes contain information in the form of DNA, which tells cells what to do and when to act.

glomerular filtration rate: A measure of the ability of the kidneys to filter and eliminate waste products from the body.

glomeruli: The network of tiny blood vessels in the kidneys through which blood is filtered and waste materials are removed.

glucagon: A hormone, made by the pancreas, that raises the level of glucose in the blood.

glucose: A simple sugar, present in the blood, that is the body's main energy source.

glucose tolerance test: A blood test that can help identify diabetes. A blood sample is taken after an overnight fast and before the individual has eaten in the morning. The person then drinks a high-glucose liquid, and a second and third blood sample are taken one and two hours later.

glycation: A biological process in which sugar molecules bind to protein molecules, which cause the latter molecules to lose their ability to function. Glycation leads to the development of advanced glycation end products.

glycogen: A substance that serves as the main source of stored energy in the body. It is composed of sugars, is stored in the liver and muscles, and is released into the bloodstream as needed.

hemoglobin A_{1c} (Hb A_{1c}): The component of red blood cells that transports oxygen to the cells and sometimes binds (glycates) with glucose. The more excess glucose you have in your blood, the more hemoglobin gets glycated. A Hb A_{1c} test measures the percentage of A_{1c} in the blood. Because glucose stays attached to hemoglobin for the life of the cell (about 120 days), the Hb A_{1c} test gives you the average of your blood glucose level for that time period. In people without diabetes, about 5 percent of their hemoglobin is glycated; for people with prediabetes or diabetes, that percentage is higher.

hyperglycemia: A condition in which blood glucose levels are abnormally high. Signs and symptoms include excessive thirst, dry mouth, and frequent urination. It is a sign that diabetes is out of control.

hyperinsulinism: A condition in which the level of insulin in the blood is abnormally high.

hypoglycemia: A condition in which blood glucose level is abnormally low. Signs and symptoms include shakiness, headache, blurry vision, hunger, nervousness, sweating, and weakness.

impaired glucose tolerance: A state in which blood glucose levels are higher than normal but not high enough to qualify as a diagnosis of diabetes; that is, a range of 100 to 126 mg/dL, which is the range assigned to prediabetes.

incretin mimetic: A class of drugs that mimics the effects of the hormones naturally secreted by the intestines. These drugs assist the body in making more insulin.

insulin: A hormone manufactured by the beta cells of the pancreas. Insulin helps the body use glucose for energy. When the pancreas cannot produce enough insulin, synthetic or recombinant DNA insulin, available as a prescription, can be injected.

insulin resistance: A condition in which the body produces insulin but is unable to respond to it properly. Insulin resistance can be associated with high blood pressure, high cholesterol and/or triglyceride levels, being overweight, and aging.

lactose: A type of sugar found in milk and milk products.

lipid: A general term for fat. Both cholesterol and triglycerides are lipids. The body stores lipids as energy and burns them when needed.

macrovascular disease: Any disease that affects the large blood vessels and is characterized by an accumulation of fat and blood clots in those vessels. The three types of macrovascular disease are cerebrovascular disease, coronary disease, and peripheral vascular disease.

metformin: The generic name for an oral antidiabetic medication (trade name Glucophage) that decreases the amount of glucose manufactured by the liver and helps make the body's cells more sensitive to insulin.

mg/dL: Milligrams per deciliter. This is the term used to describe how much glucose is present in a specific amount of blood.

microvascular disease: A condition in which the walls of the smallest blood vessels become abnormally thick and weak. This causes them to leak/bleed and interferes with blood flow, which in turn damages specific areas of the body, especially the eyes, kidneys, and the coverings (sheaths) of the nerves.

myocardial infarction: A condition in which the blood flow to the heart muscle is interrupted because of blocked or narrowed blood vessels. A myocardial infarction is also known as a heart attack.

nephropathy: A type of kidney disease in which the small blood vessels or the glomeruli (units in the kidneys that clean the blood) are damaged.

neuropathy: A disease of the nervous system in which the nerves are damaged, causing a loss of feeling. The most common type of neuropathy is peripheral, which mainly affects the feet and legs.

oxidative stress: A condition in which the production of free radicals exceeds the activity of antioxidants, which attempt to destroy them or render them inactive.

pancreas: An organ located behind the lower part of the stomach that manufactures insulin (made by beta cells), glucagon (made by alpha cells), enzymes that aid in digestion, and other substances.

peripheral neuropathy: Nerve damage that most often affects the feet and legs, causing numbness, tingling sensation, and/or pain.

phenotypic nutrition: The use of specific nutrients that have specific, known biochemical and genetic effects to help prevent disease.

polyphenols: Substances found in many plants. Polyphenols give some flowers, vegetables, and fruits their color and are excellent sources of antioxidants. They may also have some anticancer properties.

postprandial blood glucose: A blood sample taken one to two hours after eating to identify the amount of glucose in the blood.

retinopathy: A disease of the small blood vessels in the retina of the eye.

sulfonylureas: A class of oral medications used to treat high blood glucose levels. They achieve this by helping the pancreas make more insulin and by helping the body make optimal use of the insulin it does make.

thiazolidinediones: A class of oral medication that helps reduce blood glucose by making the body's cells more sensitive to insulin.

triglyceride: A type of fat found in the blood. It is removed from the blood by insulin.

Suggested Reading List

Chaitow, Leon. *Thorson's Guide to Amino Acids*. London: HarperCollins, 1991.

Cousens, Gabriel. *Depression-Free for Life*. New York: HarperCollins, 2000.

Edelstein, Michael. *Three Minute Therapy*. Aurora, CO: Glenbridge Publishers, 1997.

Eden, Donna and David Feinstein. *Energy Medicine: Balancing Your Body's Energies for Optimum Health, Joy and Vitality*. New York: Penguin, 2000.

Ellis, Albert. *Feeling Better, Getting Better, Staying Better: Profound Self-Help Therapy for Your Emotions*. Atascadero, CA: Impact Publishers, 2001.

Heriza, Nirmala. *Dr. Yoga: A Complete Guide to the Medical Benefits of Yoga*. New York: PenguinTarcher, 2004.

Hobsday, Richard. *The Healing Sun: Sunlight and Health in the 21st Century*. New York: Findhorn, 2000.

Jackson, Richard and Amy Tenderich. *Know Your Numbers, Outlive Your Diabetes: 5 Essential Health Factors You Can Master to Enjoy a Long and Healthy Life*. New York: Marlowe & Company, 2006.

Kabat-Zinn, Jon. *Mindfulness Meditation*. Niles, IL: Nightingale Conant, 2002.

Katz, David. *The Flavor Point Diet: The Delicious, Breakthrough Plan to Turn Off Your Hunger and Lose the Weight for Good.* Emmaus, PA: Rodale, 2005.

Lazarus, Arnold. *Don't Believe It for a Minute: Forty Toxic Ideas That Are Driving You Crazy.* Atascadero, CA: Impact Publishers, 1993.

Lazarus, Arnold. *The 60-Second Shrink: 101 Strategies for Staying Sane in a Crazy World.* Atascadero, CA: Impact Publishers, 1997.

Liberman, Jacob. *Light: Medicine of the Future.* Rochester, VT: Bear & Company, 1990.

Napier, Kristine. *The Omega-3 Advantage.* New York: Barnes & Noble, 2003.

Rolls, Barbara. *The Volumetrics Eating Plan: Techniques and Recipes for Feeling Full on Fewer Calories.* New York: Harper, 2007.

Rolls, Barbara and Robert A. Barnett. *The Volumetrics Weight-Control Plan.* New York: HarperTorch, 2002.

Ross, Julia. *The Mood Cure.* New York: Penguin Putnam, 2002.

Schachter, Michael B. *What Your Doctor May* Not *Tell You about Depression.* New York: Warner, 2006.

Spanek, John M. *No More Diabetes: How Yoga Saved My Life.* PublishAmerica, 2004 (self-published).

Stoll, Andrew I. *The Omega-3 Connection.* New York: Simon & Schuster, 2001.

Surwit, Richard S. *The Mind Body Diabetes Revolution.* New York: Free Press, 2004.

Thakur, Bharat. *Yoga for Diabetes Relief.* New Delhi, India: Wisdom Tree, 2007.

Weintraub, Amy. *Yoga for Depression: A Compassionate Guide to Relieving Suffering Through Yoga.* New York: Broadway Books, 2003.

Weiss, Brian L. *Meditation.* Carlsbad, CA: Hay House Inc., 2002.

Resources

Alt-Diabetes-Support
www.alt-support-diabetes.org
An online support group that offers three forums: newsgroup, IRC chat room, and Web page.

American Diabetes Association (ADA)
1701 N Beauregard St.
Alexandria, VA 22311
800-342-2383 (National Call Center)
www.diabetes.org
The goal of this organization is to prevent and cure diabetes and to improve the lives of those who have the disease.

CDC Diabetes Public Health Resource
www.cdc.gov/diabetes/
Provides information for professionals and the general public about diabetes, including research, statistics, and educational publications.

Daily Strength

www.dailystrength.org

This is the main page for this comprehensive health network. Free registration; sign up to be part of the type 2 diabetes support community.

Defeat Diabetes

www.defeatdiabetes.org/self_management/text.asp?id= Diabetes_Support_Gro

List of diabetes support groups and education programs by state.

Diabetes Care Journal

http://care.diabetesjournals.org

Online access to *Diabetes Care* and *Diabetes* journals, as well as other information.

Diabetic Mommy

www.diabeticmommy.com

Support for women who are diabetic and pregnant or who plan to become pregnant. Support for dealing with the complications of pregnancy and childbirth. Offers information, networking, online magazine, message boards.

Health Boards

www.healthboards.com

A diabetes support Web site that has partnered with WebMD. Registration is free.

Life Extension Foundation

health advisors: 800-226-2370

member care: 800-678-8989

www.lef.org

Life Extension Foundation has a twenty-seven-year history of providing important health and wellness information that emphasizes an evidence-based approach to prevention and treatment. Its Web site maintains thousands of pages of freely available reference material on every health, wellness, and disease topic imaginable.

National Diabetes Education Program (NDEP)
1 Diabetes Way
Bethesda, MD 20892-3560
800-438-5383
www.ndep.nih.gov
The goal of the NDEP is to improve the treatment and prognosis of diabetics, to promote early diagnosis, and to prevent or delay the onset of diabetes.

National Diabetes Information Clearinghouse (NDIC)
http://diabetes.niddk.nih.gov/dm/pubs/overview/index.htm
The mission of the NDIC is to increase knowledge and understanding about diabetes among the general public, patients, and health-care professionals.

National Institute of Diabetes and Digestive and Kidney Diseases
www.niddk.nih.gov/
Provides information for the general public and patients on research, clinical studies, news, and events.

Index

About the Author

For decades, Steven V. Joyal, M.D., has pursued cutting-edge interdisciplinary research in metabolic disease and endocrinology as they impact obesity as well as direct clinical work with diabetes. As a director of endocrinology and metabolism research within the pharmaceutical industry, Dr. Joyal headed a multidisciplinary research team working on drugs to treat diabetes and related conditions. He was also directly involved in the development of sibutramine (Meridia), one of only two drugs approved by the FDA for the long-term treatment of obesity. In 2005, Dr. Joyal joined the Life Extension Foundation as vice president of scientific affairs and medical development, where he is responsible for all scientific and medical research activities. He frequently lectures on the nutritional management of metabolic syndrome (prediabetes) and believes that natural supplements such as chromium (well known but little used), lipoic acid, magnesium, clove oil, bilberry, and gymnema can improve glucose metabolism and increase insulin sensitivity. He lectures about managing diabetes through weight loss at international medical conferences, has published several scholarly articles on strategies and treatments for obesity/prediabetes in peer-reviewed journals, and has been interviewed by numerous health radio shows and online health publications. He earned his medical degree from Brown University and is board certified in internal medicine.